Introduction

In a world where fad diets and extreme eating plans dominate the health and wellness landscape, have you ever wondered if there's a simpler, more sustainable way to transform your eating habits? What if the key to lasting dietary change isn't found in drastic measures, but in the power of small, consistent actions?

Welcome to "Bite-Sized Habits: Transforming Your Diet One Meal at a Time," a groundbreaking approach to nutrition that challenges the conventional wisdom of radical diet overhauls. This book is your guide to revolutionizing your relationship with food, one tiny habit at a time. In the pages that follow, you'll discover how seemingly insignificant changes can compound into remarkable results, reshaping your diet and, ultimately, your life.

For decades, we've been bombarded with conflicting nutrition advice, each new trend promising miraculous results. Yet, despite our best efforts, many of us find ourselves trapped in a cycle of yo-yo dieting, frustrated by temporary successes followed by inevitable relapses. The reason? Traditional diets often demand too much, too soon, setting us up for failure before we've even begun. But what if there was a better way?

This book introduces a fresh perspective on dietary change, one that aligns with the latest research in behavioral psychology and neuroscience. By harnessing the power of habit formation and the science of incremental progress, "Bite-Sized Habits" offers a roadmap to sustainable, long-term success in achieving your nutrition goals. Rather than advocating for sweeping changes that are difficult to maintain, we'll explore how small, manageable adjustments to your daily routines can lead to profound transformations in your eating patterns and overall health.

What sets "Bite-Sized Habits" apart from other nutrition books is its emphasis on practicality and personalization. Instead of prescribing a one-size-fits-all approach, this book provides you with the tools to create a tailored plan that fits seamlessly into your unique lifestyle. We recognize that lasting change doesn't come from following someone else's rigid rules, but from developing habits that resonate with your individual needs, preferences, and circumstances.

Throughout this journey, we'll delve into several key themes that form the foundation of the bite-sized habits approach. First, we'll explore the science of habit formation, uncovering the neurological processes that drive our behaviors and learning how to harness them for positive change. You'll gain insight into the habit loop – the cue, routine, and reward cycle that shapes our actions – and discover how to rewire it in your favor.

Next, we'll focus on the power of mindfulness in eating. In our fast-paced world, it's all too easy to eat on autopilot, disconnected from the experience of nourishing our bodies. We'll explore techniques for bringing awareness back to the dining table, helping you rediscover the joy of eating while naturally regulating portion sizes and food choices.

Another crucial theme is the importance of balanced nutrition. Rather than demonizing entire food groups or promoting extreme restrictions, we'll take a holistic approach to understanding the role of various nutrients in supporting overall health. You'll learn how to create meals that not only satisfy your taste buds but also provide your body with the diverse range of nutrients it needs to thrive.

We'll also tackle the often-overlooked psychological aspects of eating. Many of us have complex emotional relationships with food, using it as a source of comfort, celebration, or stress relief. By addressing these underlying patterns and developing healthier coping mechanisms, you'll be better equipped to make conscious choices about when, what, and how much to eat.

Lastly, we'll emphasize the importance of sustainability and long-term thinking in your nutrition journey. Instead of quick fixes or temporary solutions, we'll focus on building habits that can last a lifetime. This includes strategies for navigating social situations, dealing with setbacks, and adapting your habits as your life circumstances change.

"Bite-Sized Habits" is written for anyone who has ever struggled with their eating habits and is ready for a more effective, less stressful approach to dietary change. Whether you're a busy professional looking to improve your energy levels, a parent trying to set a good example for your children, or simply someone who wants to feel better in your body, this book offers valuable insights and practical strategies.

If you've tried and failed at diets in the past, feeling discouraged or overwhelmed by the prospect of change, this book is especially for you. We'll show you how to break down your goals into manageable steps, celebrating small victories along the way and building the confidence to tackle bigger challenges.

For those who consider themselves nutrition-savvy but struggle with consistency, "Bite-Sized Habits" provides a fresh perspective on implementing knowledge into daily practice. You'll learn how to bridge the gap between knowing what to do and actually doing it, turning good intentions into ingrained habits.

Even if you're generally satisfied with your diet but are looking to fine-tune certain aspects, this book offers advanced strategies for optimizing your nutrition and exploring new approaches to healthy eating.

By the time you finish reading "Bite-Sized Habits," you'll have gained a comprehensive toolkit for transforming your diet. You'll understand the science behind habit formation and be able to apply it to create lasting change in your eating patterns. Armed with practical strategies for mindful eating, portion control, and balanced meal planning, you'll feel empowered to make healthier choices without feeling deprived or overwhelmed.

You'll develop the skills to navigate challenging situations, from busy workdays to social gatherings, without derailing your progress. More importantly, you'll cultivate a positive, growth-oriented mindset that allows you to approach your nutrition journey with curiosity and self-compassion rather than judgment and restriction.

This book will teach you how to listen to your body's signals, helping you distinguish between true hunger and emotional eating. You'll learn to enjoy food more fully while naturally gravitating towards choices that nourish your body and support your health goals. As you implement the bite-sized habits, you may find that your energy levels increase, your mood stabilizes, and your overall sense of well-being improves.

Beyond the individual benefits, the principles you'll learn in this book can positively impact those around you. As you model healthier eating habits, you may inspire friends and family to make positive changes in their own lives. For parents, the strategies in this book offer a way to cultivate healthy attitudes towards food in your children, setting them up for a lifetime of good nutrition.

One of the most valuable outcomes of reading "Bite-Sized Habits" is the development of a flexible, adaptable approach to healthy eating. Rather than rigid rules that crumble in the face of real-life challenges, you'll have a set of principles and strategies that can evolve with you as your life circumstances change. This resilience ensures that your healthy habits can withstand the test of time, supporting you through different phases of life.

As you progress through the book, you'll find that the bite-sized habits approach extends beyond just nutrition. The principles of incremental change and consistent action can be applied to various aspects of your life, from fitness to personal development. You may discover a renewed sense of control and optimism as you realize that significant life changes are within your reach, one small step at a time.

"Bite-Sized Habits" is more than just a nutrition guide; it's an invitation to reimagine your relationship with food and, by extension, with yourself. It challenges the notion that dramatic changes are necessary for meaningful results, instead showing you the extraordinary power of small, consistent actions.

As you embark on this journey, remember that transformation doesn't happen overnight. It's the result of countless small decisions, each one building upon the last. This book will show you how to make those decisions count, guiding you towards a healthier, more balanced way of eating that feels natural and sustainable.

Are you ready to leave behind the frustration of fad diets and embrace a more intuitive, enjoyable approach to nutrition? Are you prepared to discover the profound impact that tiny changes can have on your overall health and well-being? Then it's time to dive into the world of bite-sized habits.

In the chapters that follow, we'll break down the process of dietary change into manageable, actionable steps. We'll explore how to assess your current eating habits, set realistic goals, and gradually implement new behaviors that align with your vision of health. You'll learn practical strategies for mindful eating, portion control, and meal planning, as well as techniques for overcoming common obstacles and setbacks.

We'll delve into the specifics of creating balanced meals, from quick and nutritious breakfasts to satisfying dinners that please the whole family. You'll discover how to navigate social eating situations, manage cravings, and find joy in nourishing your body. We'll also explore the important connection between nutrition and physical activity, helping you create a holistic approach to health that encompasses both diet and exercise.

Throughout the book, you'll find real-life examples, practical exercises, and reflection prompts that will help you apply the concepts to your own life. These interactive elements are designed to deepen your understanding and facilitate the process of habit formation, ensuring that the knowledge you gain translates into tangible changes in your daily routines.

As we near the end of our journey, we'll look at advanced strategies for those who want to take their healthy eating habits to the next level. We'll explore topics like plant-based eating, intermittent fasting, and intuitive eating, providing you with a glimpse into various nutritional approaches that you might choose to incorporate into your lifestyle.

Finally, we'll discuss how to maintain your new habits over the long term, adapting them as your life evolves and continuing to grow in your nutritional knowledge. You'll learn how to become a lifelong student of health and nutrition, always open to new information but grounded in the fundamental principles of the bite-sized habits approach.

So, are you ready to transform your diet, one small change at a time? Are you prepared to discover the power of bite-sized habits and their potential to revolutionize not just your eating patterns, but your entire approach to health and well-being? Then turn the page, and let's begin this exciting journey towards a healthier, happier you. The path to lasting dietary change starts here, with the very next bite you take.

Chapter 1: The Power of Tiny Changes

The journey of a thousand miles begins with a single step. This ancient wisdom, attributed to the Chinese philosopher Lao Tzu, encapsulates the essence of transformative change. In the realm of nutrition and dietary habits, this principle holds particularly true. The power of tiny changes lies not in their immediate impact, but in their cumulative effect over time. It is this compounding effect that forms the foundation of the bite-sized habits approach to transforming your diet.

Consider for a moment the last time you attempted to overhaul your entire diet in one sweeping change. Perhaps you decided to cut out all carbohydrates, or committed to eating only raw foods. How long did this drastic change last? For most people, such radical shifts are unsustainable, leading to frustration, guilt, and ultimately, a return to old habits. This is because our brains are wired to resist sudden, large-scale changes. Instead, they thrive on small, consistent adjustments that can be easily integrated into our daily routines.

The compounding effect of small habits is akin to compound interest in finance. Just as a small amount of money invested regularly can grow into a substantial sum over time, tiny changes in our eating habits can lead to significant improvements in our overall health and well-being. For instance, replacing your afternoon soda with a glass of water might seem inconsequential in the moment. However, over the course of a year, this simple swap could result in consuming 50,000 fewer calories and avoiding over 3,000 teaspoons of sugar. This single, seemingly minor change could lead to weight loss, improved dental health, better hydration, and reduced risk of type 2 diabetes.

Dr. BJ Fogg, a behavior scientist at Stanford University, emphasizes the power of tiny habits in his research. He states, "To create a new habit, you must first simplify the behavior. Make it tiny, even ridiculous. A good tiny behavior is easy to do — and fast." This principle is at the heart of the bite-sized habits approach to nutrition. By breaking down the complex goal of "eating healthier" into small, manageable actions, we set ourselves up for success.

Traditional diets often fail because they rely on willpower and motivation, both of which are finite resources. When we attempt to make sweeping changes to our eating habits, we quickly deplete these resources, leading to what psychologists call "decision fatigue." This state of mental exhaustion makes it increasingly difficult to make good choices, often resulting in a return to old, comfortable habits.

Moreover, traditional diets frequently focus on restriction and deprivation, which can trigger a psychological response known as the "scarcity mindset." When we feel that certain foods are off-limits, we tend to fixate on them, increasing our cravings and making it more likely that we'll eventually give in and overindulge. This cycle of restriction and bingeing not only undermines our dietary goals but can also lead to an unhealthy relationship with food.

Another reason why traditional diets often fail is their one-size-fits-all approach. Every individual has unique nutritional needs, food preferences, and lifestyle factors that influence their eating habits. A diet that works well for one person may be completely unsustainable for another. The bite-sized habits approach, on the other hand, allows for personalization and flexibility, making it adaptable to various lifestyles and dietary requirements.

The introduction to the bite-sized habits approach marks a paradigm shift in how we think about dietary change. Instead of focusing on drastic measures or quick fixes, this method emphasizes the power of incremental improvements. It's about making small, consistent changes that align with your personal goals and lifestyle, gradually building a foundation for lasting health and wellness.

At its core, the bite-sized habits approach is rooted in behavioral psychology and neuroscience. It leverages our understanding of how habits are formed and maintained in the brain. By focusing on one small change at a time, we reduce the cognitive load associated with behavior change, making it easier for our brains to adapt and create new neural pathways.

The beauty of this approach lies in its simplicity and accessibility. You don't need special equipment, expensive meal plans, or a complete lifestyle overhaul to get started. Instead, you begin with a single, manageable change – perhaps drinking a glass of water before each meal, or adding an extra serving of vegetables to your dinner plate. As this new habit becomes ingrained, you can build upon it, gradually expanding your repertoire of healthy eating behaviors.

Dr. James Clear, author of "Atomic Habits," explains this concept eloquently: "Habits are the compound interest of self-improvement. The same way that money multiplies through compound interest, the effects of your habits multiply as you repeat them." This compounding effect is what makes the bite-sized habits approach so powerful. Each small change you make builds upon the last, creating a snowball effect of positive transformation in your diet and overall health.

It's important to note that the bite-sized habits approach is not about perfection, but progress. It acknowledges that setbacks and slip-ups are a normal part of any change process. Rather than viewing these moments as failures, they are seen as opportunities for learning and adjustment. This mindset shift is crucial for long-term success, as it fosters resilience and prevents the all-or-nothing thinking that often derails traditional diets.

The bite-sized habits approach also aligns well with the concept of mindfulness in eating. By focusing on small, deliberate changes, we become more aware of our food choices and eating patterns. This increased awareness can lead to a more intuitive relationship with food, where we learn to listen to our body's hunger and fullness cues, and make choices that truly nourish us.

As we delve deeper into the bite-sized habits approach, it's crucial to understand that this method is not just about changing what you eat, but also how you think about food and nutrition. It's about cultivating a growth mindset around your eating habits, believing that you can improve and evolve over time. This positive outlook can have far-reaching effects beyond just your diet, influencing other areas of your life where small, consistent changes can lead to significant improvements.

The power of tiny changes extends beyond the individual level. As you begin to implement bite-sized habits in your own life, you may find that your positive choices influence those around you. Your family members might become curious about your new eating habits, or your colleagues might be inspired by your healthy lunch choices. In this way, the ripple effect of your small changes can contribute to a broader culture of health and wellness.

It's worth noting that the bite-sized habits approach is not a quick fix or a short-term solution. It's a sustainable, long-term strategy for improving your nutrition and overall health. Unlike crash diets or extreme eating plans that promise rapid results, this method focuses on gradual, lasting change. It acknowledges that true transformation takes time and patience, but the results are far more enduring.

As we move forward in this book, we'll explore various aspects of nutrition and healthy eating through the lens of bite-sized habits. We'll delve into the science of habit formation, learn how to assess our current eating patterns, and discover practical strategies for implementing small, meaningful changes in our daily lives. Each chapter will build upon the last, providing you with a comprehensive toolkit for transforming your diet one meal at a time.

Remember, the journey to better nutrition is not a straight line. There will be ups and downs, successes and challenges. But by embracing the power of tiny changes, you're setting yourself up for long-term success. As the renowned nutrition expert Michael Pollan once said, "Eat food. Not too much. Mostly plants." This simple advice encapsulates the essence of healthy eating, and with the bite-sized habits approach, you'll learn how to implement these principles in a way that works for you.

As we conclude this chapter on the power of tiny changes, it's important to reflect on the key takeaways. We've learned that small, consistent changes can lead to significant improvements in our diet and overall health. We've understood why traditional diets often fail and how the bite-sized habits approach offers a more sustainable alternative. We've explored the concept of compound effect in habit formation and how it applies to our eating behaviors.

In the next chapter, we'll delve deeper into the science of habit formation. We'll explore the neurological basis of habits, understand the habit loop of cue, routine, and reward, and examine how these principles specifically apply to our eating behaviors. This foundation will be crucial as we begin to implement bite-sized habits in our own lives, paving the way for lasting positive change in our nutrition journey.

Chapter 2: The Science of Habit Formation

As we delve deeper into the journey of transforming our diet through bite-sized habits, it's crucial to understand the underlying mechanisms that drive our behaviors. The science of habit formation provides us with valuable insights into why we do what we do, and more importantly, how we can reshape our actions to align with our health goals. This chapter will explore the neurological basis of habits, unpack the components of the habit loop, and examine how these principles specifically apply to our eating behaviors.

The human brain is a marvel of efficiency, constantly seeking ways to conserve energy and streamline processes. Habits are one of the brain's most powerful tools for achieving this efficiency. Neuroscientists have discovered that habitual behaviors are deeply ingrained in our neural pathways, allowing us to perform routine actions with minimal mental effort. This automation frees up cognitive resources for more complex tasks, but it also means that once a habit is formed, it can be challenging to alter.

At the core of habit formation lies the basal ganglia, a group of subcortical nuclei that play a crucial role in learning, motor control, and executive functions. When we repeat a behavior consistently, the basal ganglia begin to encode this action as a habit, creating a neural shortcut that allows us to perform the behavior automatically. This process is known as chunking, where a complex set of actions is compressed into a single routine.

Dr. Ann Graybiel, a neuroscientist at MIT, explains the power of this process: "The brain's ability to chunk actions together into a single routine is a fundamental aspect of learning and allows us to carry out complex behaviors without conscious thought." This chunking mechanism is what allows us to perform intricate tasks like driving a car or typing on a keyboard without actively thinking about each individual movement.

However, the same neural mechanisms that make habits so efficient can also make them stubbornly resistant to change. Once a habit is formed, it creates a strong neural pathway in the brain. Trying to break this habit essentially means forging a new neural pathway, which requires consistent effort and repetition. This is why many people struggle to change their dietary habits, even when they have a strong desire to do so.

Understanding the neurological basis of habits is just the first step. To truly harness the power of habit formation for dietary change, we need to examine the structure of habits themselves. This brings us to the concept of the habit loop, a framework popularized by Charles Duhigg in his book "The Power of Habit."

The habit loop consists of three key components: the cue, the routine, and the reward. The cue is the trigger that initiates the habit, the routine is the behavior itself, and the reward is the positive reinforcement that tells our brain the behavior is worth remembering and repeating. This loop is the foundation of all habits, including those related to our eating behaviors.

Let's consider a common eating habit through the lens of the habit loop. The cue might be feeling stressed after a long day at work. The routine is reaching for a bag of chips and mindlessly snacking while watching TV. The reward is the temporary relief from stress and the pleasurable taste sensation. Over time, this loop becomes automated, and we find ourselves repeating this behavior whenever we feel stressed, often without even realizing it.

The power of the habit loop lies in its ability to create a craving. As we repeat a habit loop, our brain begins to anticipate the reward even before we complete the routine. This anticipation creates a subtle neurological craving that drives us to perform the routine whenever we encounter the cue. In the case of our stress-eating example, we might start craving chips as soon as we feel stressed, even before we've had a chance to consciously decide what to eat.

Understanding this loop is crucial for changing our eating habits. By identifying the cues that trigger our unhealthy eating routines and the rewards we're seeking, we can begin to reshape these habits. The key is not to try to eliminate the habit entirely, but to replace the routine with a healthier alternative that provides a similar reward.

For instance, in our stress-eating example, we might replace the routine of eating chips with a short meditation session or a brisk walk. If we consistently pair this new routine with the same cue (feeling stressed) and ensure it provides a similar reward (stress relief), we can gradually rewire our habit loop. Over time, our brain will begin to crave the new, healthier routine when we encounter the stress cue.

It's important to note that changing habits is rarely a linear process. Dr. Wendy Wood, a psychologist at the University of Southern California who has extensively studied habit formation, emphasizes that habit change often involves a period of conscious effort before the new behavior becomes automatic. "Habits form through repetition," she explains. "The more consistently you perform a behavior in a given context, the more automatic it becomes."

This insight is particularly relevant when it comes to our eating behaviors. Many of our food-related habits are deeply ingrained, shaped by years of repetition and influenced by a complex interplay of biological, psychological, and environmental factors. Our food choices are not just about sustenance; they're often tied to emotions, social situations, and cultural norms.

Consider how habits shape our daily eating patterns. Many of us have a habitual breakfast routine, reaching for the same foods each morning without much thought. Our lunch habits might be influenced by workplace norms or time constraints. Dinner routines often revolve around family schedules or social commitments. These habitual patterns can work for or against our nutrition goals, depending on the specific behaviors we've automated.

Moreover, our eating habits are often intertwined with other lifestyle habits. For example, the habit of watching TV after dinner might be paired with the habit of snacking, even when we're not hungry. The habit of staying up late might lead to late-night eating, disrupting our natural hunger and fullness cues. By recognizing these interconnected habit loops, we can begin to address our eating behaviors more holistically.

One of the challenges in changing eating habits is the immediate and potent reward that food often provides. Highly palatable foods, particularly those high in sugar, salt, and fat, activate the brain's reward centers, releasing dopamine and creating a pleasurable sensation. This immediate reward can override our long-term health goals, making it difficult to resist temptation in the moment.

Dr. Nora Volkow, Director of the National Institute on Drug Abuse, has conducted extensive research on the neurobiology of eating behaviors. Her work has shown that for some individuals, certain foods can trigger brain responses similar to those seen in drug addiction. "The same brain circuits that are affected by drugs of abuse are also activated by foods that are high in sugar, fat, and salt," she explains. This doesn't mean that food is addictive in the same way as drugs, but it does highlight the powerful influence that habitual eating patterns can have on our brain chemistry.

Understanding this neurological perspective can help us approach habit change with more compassion and patience. It explains why simply trying to use willpower to resist unhealthy foods often fails in the long run. Instead, we need to work with our brain's reward system, gradually reshaping our habits to find healthier sources of pleasure and satisfaction.

As we conclude this exploration of the science behind habit formation, it's clear that our eating behaviors are deeply influenced by neurological processes and habitual patterns. This knowledge forms the foundation for the bite-sized habits approach to dietary change. By understanding how habits are formed and maintained in the brain, we can develop more effective strategies for transforming our eating behaviors.

In the next chapter, we'll build on this scientific foundation by turning our attention inward. We'll explore methods for assessing our current eating habits, identifying the specific cues, routines, and rewards that drive our food-related behaviors. This self-reflection is a crucial step in the process of habit change, allowing us to pinpoint areas for improvement and develop targeted strategies for implementing healthier habits. Armed with both scientific understanding and personal insight, we'll be well-equipped to begin the journey of transforming our diet, one small habit at a time.

Chapter 3: Assessing Your Current Eating Habits

As we embark on the journey of transforming our diet through bite-sized habits, it's crucial to first take stock of where we currently stand. Our eating habits, like any other behaviors, are deeply ingrained and often operate on autopilot. To effectively change these habits, we must first bring them into our conscious awareness. This chapter will guide you through the process of self-reflection, help you identify trigger foods and situations, and recognize emotional eating patterns that may be influencing your dietary choices.

Self-reflection exercises are an invaluable tool in understanding our relationship with food. These exercises allow us to pause and examine our behaviors, thoughts, and feelings surrounding eating. One effective method is keeping a detailed food diary for at least a week. This involves noting not just what you eat, but also when, where, and how you feel before, during, and after eating. Dr. Brian Wansink, a renowned food psychologist, states, "The first step in making any change is to become aware of our current behaviors. A food diary can reveal patterns we never knew existed."

As you maintain your food diary, pay close attention to the circumstances surrounding your meals and snacks. Are you eating at regular intervals, or do you tend to graze throughout the day? Do you eat while distracted by work, television, or your phone? These observations can provide valuable insights into your eating habits and help identify areas for improvement.

Another crucial aspect of self-reflection is examining your emotional state in relation to food. Many of us turn to food for comfort, stress relief, or as a reward. While there's nothing inherently wrong with finding pleasure in food, emotional eating can often lead to overconsumption and poor food choices. Dr. Jane Ogden, a professor of health psychology, explains, "Emotional eating is a common coping mechanism, but it's important to recognize when we're eating to satisfy emotional needs rather than physical hunger."

To explore your emotional eating patterns, consider keeping an "emotion and food" log alongside your food diary. Each time you eat, note your emotional state and the intensity of that emotion on a scale of 1 to 10. Over time, you may start to see correlations between certain emotions and specific eating behaviors. For instance, you might notice that you tend to reach for sugary snacks when feeling anxious or that you eat larger portions when stressed.

Identifying trigger foods and situations is another crucial step in assessing your current eating habits. Trigger foods are those that you find difficult to resist or control your intake of once you start eating them. These can vary greatly from person to person. For some, it might be potato chips or cookies, while for others, it could be seemingly healthy foods like nuts or fruit.

To identify your trigger foods, review your food diary and look for items that you tend to overeat or that leave you feeling out of control. Pay attention to the context in which these foods appear. Are there certain times of day, locations, or social situations where you're more likely to indulge in these foods? Understanding these patterns can help you develop strategies to manage your consumption of trigger foods more effectively.

Situations that trigger overeating or poor food choices are equally important to identify. Common triggers include social gatherings, work stress, boredom, or even specific locations like the couch in front of the TV. Dr. Judith Beck, a cognitive behavioral therapist specializing in weight management, notes, "Once you identify your challenging situations, you can prepare in advance and develop coping strategies to navigate them more successfully."

As you engage in these self-reflection exercises, it's crucial to approach the process with curiosity and compassion rather than judgment. Remember, the goal is not to criticize your current habits but to understand them better. This understanding will serve as the foundation for the positive changes you'll be making in the coming chapters.

Recognizing emotional eating patterns is a particularly important aspect of assessing your current eating habits. Emotional eating refers to the tendency to use food to cope with emotions, rather than to satisfy physical hunger. This pattern can be particularly challenging to overcome because it often provides short-term relief or comfort, even though it may lead to feelings of guilt or shame afterwards.

To delve deeper into your emotional eating patterns, consider the following questions: Do you find yourself reaching for food when you're not physically hungry? Do you use food as a reward or to celebrate? Do you eat to alleviate boredom, loneliness, or stress? Answering these questions honestly can help you identify the emotional triggers that lead to unhealthy eating behaviors.

Dr. Linda Craighead, author of "The Appetite Awareness Workbook," suggests, "By becoming more aware of the connection between our emotions and our eating behaviors, we can start to develop alternative coping strategies that don't involve food." This might involve finding other ways to self-soothe, such as taking a walk, practicing deep breathing exercises, or calling a friend when you're feeling stressed or upset.

It's also important to pay attention to the types of foods you turn to when eating emotionally. Often, emotional eating involves consuming high-calorie, high-fat, or high-sugar foods that provide a quick but temporary mood boost. By identifying these patterns, you can start to make more conscious choices about how you respond to emotional triggers.

Another aspect of assessing your current eating habits involves examining your relationship with food on a broader level. Do you view certain foods as "good" or "bad"? Do you have rigid rules about when or what you can eat? These attitudes can often lead to an unhealthy cycle of restriction and overindulgence. As you reflect on your habits, try to notice any black-and-white thinking patterns you might have about food and eating.

It's also valuable to consider the role that your environment plays in shaping your eating habits. Our food choices are often influenced by factors such as the availability of certain foods in our home or workplace, the eating habits of those around us, and even the layout of our kitchen. Dr. Brian Wansink's research has shown that simple environmental changes, like keeping fruits and vegetables in visible and easily accessible locations, can significantly impact our food choices.

As you assess your current eating habits, don't forget to consider your meal patterns and timing. Do you tend to skip meals, particularly breakfast? Do you find yourself snacking late at night? These patterns can have a significant impact on your overall nutrition and energy levels. Registered dietitian Evelyn Tribole advises, "Regular, balanced meals can help stabilize blood sugar levels and reduce the likelihood of overeating later in the day."

It's also important to reflect on the pace at which you eat. Many of us eat quickly, often while distracted, which can lead to overconsumption and reduced satisfaction from our meals. Mindful eating expert Dr. Jan Chozen Bays suggests, "Slowing down and paying attention to the sensory experience of eating can help us feel more satisfied with less food and make meals more enjoyable."

As you go through this process of self-reflection and assessment, remember that everyone's relationship with food is unique and complex. There's no one-size-fits-all approach to healthy eating, and what works for one person may not work for another. The goal of this assessment is to gain a deeper understanding of your own patterns and behaviors, which will serve as the foundation for the positive changes you'll be making.

It's also worth noting that our eating habits don't exist in isolation. They're often deeply intertwined with other aspects of our lives, including our work, relationships, and overall lifestyle. As you reflect on your eating habits, consider how they relate to other areas of your life. For instance, do long work hours lead to rushed, unhealthy meals? Does stress in your relationships trigger emotional eating?

Dr. Michelle May, author of "Eat What You Love, Love What You Eat," emphasizes the importance of this holistic approach: "Our eating habits are just one part of our overall health and well-being. By understanding how they connect to other aspects of our lives, we can make more meaningful and sustainable changes."

As we conclude this chapter on assessing your current eating habits, it's important to remember that this is just the beginning of your journey. The insights you've gained through these self-reflection exercises will serve as a valuable roadmap as we move forward. In the next chapter, we'll build on this foundation by exploring how to set realistic nutrition goals that align with your personal values and lifestyle. This process of self-discovery and goal-setting will be crucial in creating lasting, positive changes in your eating habits.

Chapter 4: Setting Realistic Nutrition Goals

As we've explored the science behind habit formation and assessed our current eating patterns, we're now poised to take a crucial step in our journey towards healthier eating: setting realistic nutrition goals. This process is far more nuanced than simply declaring, "I want to eat better." It requires thoughtful consideration, self-awareness, and a strategic approach that aligns with our individual lifestyles and values.

SMART goal setting has long been a cornerstone of successful behavior change, and it's particularly effective when applied to dietary modifications. The acronym SMART stands for Specific, Measurable, Achievable, Relevant, and Time-bound. By framing our nutrition goals within this structure, we significantly increase our chances of success and sustainable change.

Let's begin with the 'Specific' aspect of goal setting. Rather than making a vague statement like "I want to eat healthier," a specific goal might be "I will include a serving of vegetables with every dinner." This clarity helps to focus our efforts and provides a clear target to aim for. Specificity eliminates ambiguity and gives us a concrete action to take, making it easier to track progress and maintain motivation.

The 'Measurable' component of SMART goals is crucial for nutrition objectives. It allows us to quantify our progress and know definitively whether we're achieving what we set out to do. For instance, instead of saying "I'll drink more water," a measurable goal would be "I'll drink 8 glasses of water daily." This measurability provides a sense of accomplishment as we tick off our daily water intake, reinforcing our commitment to the new habit.

'Achievable' goals are those that stretch us but remain within the realm of possibility. It's important to challenge ourselves, but setting unrealistic goals can lead to frustration and abandonment of our efforts. For example, completely eliminating sugar from one's diet overnight is likely unrealistic for most people. A more achievable goal might be to reduce added sugar intake by 25% over the course of a month. This gradual approach allows for adaptation and increases the likelihood of long-term success.

The 'Relevant' aspect of goal setting ensures that our nutrition objectives align with our broader life goals and values. This alignment is crucial for maintaining motivation and making lasting changes. For instance, if one of your core values is environmental sustainability, a relevant nutrition goal might be to incorporate more plant-based meals into your diet. This goal not only improves your health but also aligns with your environmental values, providing additional motivation.

Lastly, 'Time-bound' goals give us a sense of urgency and help prevent procrastination. Setting a deadline or timeframe for achieving our nutrition goals creates a sense of commitment and helps us prioritize our efforts. For example, "I will learn to cook three new vegetable-based dishes by the end of this month" provides a clear timeframe and a specific target to work towards.

When setting nutrition goals, it's crucial to align them with our personal values and lifestyle. This alignment ensures that our goals feel authentic and meaningful to us, rather than imposed from external sources. Consider what truly matters to you. Is it having more energy to play with your children? Reducing your risk of chronic diseases? Feeling more confident in your body? Whatever your personal motivations, let them guide your goal-setting process.

It's also important to recognize that our lifestyles play a significant role in shaping our eating habits. A busy executive with frequent business dinners will have different challenges and opportunities compared to a stay-at-home parent preparing meals for a family. Acknowledging these realities and crafting goals that work within the constraints of our lives is crucial for success. For instance, the executive might set a goal to identify three healthy options on commonly visited restaurant menus, while the stay-at-home parent might focus on involving children in meal preparation to encourage healthier eating habits for the whole family.

One common pitfall in nutrition goal setting is an excessive focus on weight loss. While weight management can be a valid health concern, prioritizing health over weight loss often leads to more sustainable and positive outcomes. This shift in focus can be transformative. Instead of setting a goal to lose a certain number of pounds, consider goals that directly impact your health and well-being. For example, aiming to increase your daily fiber intake, reduce processed food consumption, or incorporate a wider variety of fruits and vegetables into your diet.

This health-focused approach has several advantages. Firstly, it encourages a more positive relationship with food and our bodies. When we focus solely on weight, we often fall into restrictive patterns that can be unsustainable and even harmful. By contrast, health-focused goals allow us to appreciate food as nourishment and to view our dietary choices as acts of self-care rather than punishment or deprivation.

Secondly, prioritizing health over weight loss often leads to more sustainable changes. Weight can fluctuate due to various factors beyond our control, potentially leading to frustration if it's our primary measure of success. Health-focused goals, on the other hand, often result in noticeable improvements in energy levels, mood, digestion, and overall well-being – changes that can be felt relatively quickly and provide ongoing motivation.

As we set our nutrition goals, it's also important to consider the concept of habit stacking, introduced by James Clear in his book "Atomic Habits." Habit stacking involves linking a new habit to an existing one, making it easier to remember and implement. For example, if you already have a habit of making coffee every morning, you might set a goal to drink a glass of water while your coffee brews. This strategy leverages existing routines to facilitate the adoption of new, healthier habits.

Another crucial aspect of setting realistic nutrition goals is to anticipate and plan for obstacles. No journey towards healthier eating is without challenges, and acknowledging this from the outset can help us develop strategies to overcome potential hurdles. For each goal you set, consider what might get in the way of achieving it. If your goal is to cook more meals at home, but you often work late, you might plan to batch cook on weekends or invest in a slow cooker for easy weeknight meals.

It's also valuable to build flexibility into our goals. Rigid, all-or-nothing thinking can be detrimental to long-term success. Instead, consider setting goals with built-in flexibility. For instance, rather than aiming to completely eliminate a certain food, you might set a goal to limit it to once a week. This approach allows for occasional indulgence without derailing your entire plan, promoting a more balanced and sustainable approach to healthy eating.

As we conclude this chapter on setting realistic nutrition goals, it's important to remember that this is a dynamic process. Our goals should evolve as we progress in our journey towards healthier eating. What seems challenging today may become second nature in a few months, allowing us to set more ambitious goals. Conversely, we may find that some goals need to be adjusted if they prove too difficult or don't align well with our lifestyle.

The key is to approach goal setting with a spirit of curiosity and self-compassion. Each goal we set, whether we achieve it fully or not, is an opportunity to learn more about ourselves and our relationship with food. As we move forward, we'll explore specific strategies for implementing these goals, starting with one of the most fundamental aspects of healthy eating: understanding the building blocks of a nutritious diet.

Chapter 5: The Building Blocks of a Healthy Diet

As we transition from setting realistic nutrition goals, it's crucial to understand the fundamental components that make up a healthy diet. This knowledge forms the foundation upon which we can build our bite-sized habits, ensuring that each small change we make contributes to overall nutritional wellbeing.

Essential nutrients and their roles

At the core of any healthy diet are the essential nutrients our bodies need to function optimally. These nutrients are categorized into six main groups: carbohydrates, proteins, fats, vitamins, minerals, and water. Each plays a vital role in maintaining our health and supporting various bodily functions.

Carbohydrates are our body's primary source of energy. They fuel our brain, muscles, and organs, enabling us to think clearly and perform physical activities. Complex carbohydrates, found in whole grains, legumes, and vegetables, are particularly beneficial as they provide sustained energy and are rich in fiber. Fiber aids in digestion, helps maintain a healthy gut microbiome, and contributes to feelings of fullness, which can assist in weight management.

Proteins are often referred to as the building blocks of life, and for good reason. They are essential for the growth and repair of tissues, the production of enzymes and hormones, and the maintenance of a healthy immune system. While animal products like meat, fish, eggs, and dairy are complete protein sources, plant-based proteins from legumes, nuts, and seeds can also provide all the necessary amino acids when consumed in varied combinations.

Fats, contrary to their often-negative reputation, are crucial for our health. They help in the absorption of fat-soluble vitamins (A, D, E, and K), provide insulation for our organs, and contribute to brain health. The key is to focus on healthy fats found in foods like avocados, nuts, seeds, and fatty fish, while limiting saturated and trans fats.

Vitamins and minerals, though needed in smaller quantities, are no less important. They act as cofactors in numerous bodily processes, from energy production to bone health. For instance, vitamin C supports our immune system and aids in collagen production, while calcium and vitamin D are crucial for strong bones and teeth. Iron is essential for oxygen transport in our blood, and potassium helps regulate blood pressure.

Water, often overlooked in discussions about nutrition, is perhaps the most critical nutrient of all. It makes up a significant portion of our body weight and is involved in virtually every bodily function. Proper hydration supports digestion, nutrient absorption, temperature regulation, and waste elimination.

Understanding these nutrients and their roles allows us to make informed choices about our diet. As Marion Nestle, professor of Nutrition, Food Studies, and Public Health at New York University, aptly puts it, "The basic principles of good diets are so simple that

I can summarize them in just ten words: eat less, move more, eat lots of fruits and vegetables."

Balanced plate model

While knowing about individual nutrients is important, applying this knowledge to create balanced meals can be challenging. This is where the balanced plate model comes in handy. This visual guide simplifies the process of creating nutritionally balanced meals and helps ensure we're getting a good mix of all essential nutrients.

The balanced plate model typically divides a plate into sections: half the plate should be filled with fruits and vegetables, a quarter with whole grains or starchy vegetables, and the remaining quarter with lean proteins. A small serving of healthy fats can be included as well.

This model is flexible and can be adapted to various dietary preferences and cultural cuisines. For instance, in a Mediterranean-style meal, the vegetable portion might include a large Greek salad, the grain section could be whole wheat pita bread, and the protein could be grilled fish with a drizzle of olive oil for healthy fats.

The beauty of the balanced plate model lies in its simplicity and adaptability. It doesn't require calorie counting or strict portion control, but rather encourages a natural balance of nutrients. By following this model, we can ensure that we're getting a good mix of carbohydrates for energy, proteins for tissue repair and satiety, and a variety of vitamins and minerals from fruits and vegetables.

Moreover, the balanced plate model naturally promotes portion control. By filling half the plate with low-calorie, nutrient-dense vegetables and fruits, we automatically limit the space available for more calorie-dense foods. This can be particularly helpful for those looking to manage their weight without feeling deprived.

Dr. Walter Willett, Professor of Epidemiology and Nutrition at Harvard T.H. Chan School of Public Health, emphasizes the importance of such an approach: "The traditional Mediterranean diet provides a great example of a healthy dietary pattern. This diet emphasizes olive oil, vegetables, fruits, nuts, beans and peas, unrefined grains, and fish. It includes only small amounts of meat and full-fat dairy products. This pattern is associated with a lower risk of chronic diseases and obesity."

Importance of variety in food choices

While the balanced plate model provides a solid framework for healthy eating, the importance of variety within this framework cannot be overstated. Consuming a wide array of foods not only ensures that we're getting all the necessary nutrients but also makes our meals more enjoyable and sustainable in the long term.

Variety in our diet serves multiple purposes. Firstly, it helps us obtain a broad spectrum of nutrients. Different foods contain different combinations of vitamins, minerals, and phytonutrients. For example, while oranges are known for their vitamin C content, bell peppers actually contain more of this vitamin per serving. By including both in our diet, along with other fruits and vegetables, we ensure a steady supply of not just vitamin C, but also other beneficial compounds unique to each food.

Secondly, dietary variety supports gut health. Our gut microbiome, the complex ecosystem of bacteria living in our digestive tract, thrives on diversity. Different types of fiber and plant compounds feed different bacterial species, promoting a more balanced and resilient microbiome. This, in turn, can have far-reaching effects on our overall health, from improved digestion to enhanced immune function and even better mental health.

Thirdly, variety in our food choices can help prevent nutritional deficiencies. While it's possible to meet our basic nutritional needs with a limited range of foods, doing so requires careful planning and leaves little room for error. By regularly rotating through a wide array of foods, we create a nutritional safety net, reducing the risk of falling short on any particular nutrient.

Moreover, variety adds interest and pleasure to our meals, which is crucial for long-term adherence to healthy eating habits. Eating the same foods day in and day out can lead to boredom and increase the likelihood of straying from our nutritional goals. On the other hand, experimenting with different foods, flavors, and cuisines can turn healthy eating into an exciting culinary adventure.

Dr. David Katz, founding director of Yale University's Yale-Griffin Prevention Research Center, emphasizes this point: "The more variable the diet, the more likely it is to be nutritionally complete. Also, variety is the spice of life, and it makes our diets more interesting and enjoyable."

Incorporating variety into our diet doesn't have to be complicated. It can be as simple as trying a new fruit or vegetable each week, experimenting with different whole grains, or exploring plant-based protein sources. Even small changes, like swapping almonds for walnuts as a snack or trying a new type of leafy green in our salads, can contribute to greater dietary diversity.

When it comes to proteins, alternating between fish, poultry, lean meats, eggs, and plant-based options like legumes and tofu not only provides different nutrient profiles but also exposes us to a range of culinary experiences. Similarly, exploring different cooking methods can transform familiar ingredients into novel meals, adding variety without necessarily introducing new foods.

It's worth noting that while variety is important, it doesn't mean we need to eat something different at every meal. Rather, it's about ensuring diversity over time. We might have our favorite breakfast that we eat most days, but vary our lunches and dinners throughout the week. The goal is to create a dietary pattern that is both nutritionally complete and enjoyable over the long term.

As we consider the building blocks of a healthy diet – essential nutrients, the balanced plate model, and the importance of variety – it becomes clear that healthy eating is not about strict limitations or depriving ourselves of the foods we love. Instead, it's about feeling great, having more energy, improving our health, and stabilizing our mood. By understanding these fundamental principles, we lay the groundwork for developing bite-sized habits that can transform our relationship with food and enhance our overall wellbeing.

As we move forward to explore mindful eating in the next chapter, remember that these building blocks form the foundation upon which all our future habits will be built. The knowledge of essential nutrients helps us make informed choices, the balanced plate model gives us a practical framework for creating healthy meals, and embracing variety ensures that our journey towards better nutrition is both effective and enjoyable. With this solid foundation, we're well-equipped to take our first steps into mindful eating, our inaugural bite-sized habit in this transformative journey.

Chapter 6: Mindful Eating: Your First Bite-Sized Habit

As we transition from understanding the building blocks of a healthy diet, we now turn our attention to the practice that will serve as the foundation for all your future dietary changes: mindful eating. This seemingly simple yet profoundly impactful habit has the power to revolutionize your relationship with food and set the stage for sustainable, long-term improvements in your nutrition.

Mindful eating is rooted in the broader concept of mindfulness, which involves being fully present and engaged in the current moment. When applied to our eating habits, this practice encourages us to bring our full attention to the experience of consuming food. It's about savoring each bite, recognizing the flavors, textures, and aromas of our meals, and tuning into our body's signals of hunger and fullness.

The importance of mindful eating cannot be overstated in our modern world of constant distractions and fast-paced lifestyles. Many of us have fallen into the habit of eating on autopilot, barely registering what we're consuming as we multitask during meals or rush through our food to get to the next task. This disconnection from our eating experience can lead to overconsumption, poor food choices, and a general lack of satisfaction from our meals.

By cultivating mindfulness around our eating habits, we can begin to reverse these trends and develop a healthier, more balanced approach to nutrition. Mindful eating allows us to derive greater pleasure from our food, potentially leading to increased satisfaction with smaller portions. It also helps us become more attuned to our body's true needs, distinguishing between physical hunger and emotional or habitual eating triggers.

One of the fundamental techniques for eating with awareness is to engage all of our senses during a meal. This means taking the time to visually appreciate the colors and presentation of our food before we begin eating. As we take our first bite, we should pay close attention to the various flavors that dance across our palate, noting the interplay of sweet, salty, sour, bitter, and umami tastes. We should also be aware of the texture of the food in our mouths, whether it's crisp, creamy, crunchy, or tender.

The sound of our food can also play a role in our eating experience. The satisfying crunch of fresh vegetables or the sizzle of a stir-fry can enhance our enjoyment and engagement with the meal. Even the aroma of our food is an important part of mindful eating. Taking a moment to inhale deeply before we begin eating can stimulate our appetite and prime our digestive system for the meal to come.

As we practice these techniques, it's important to remember that mindful eating is not about perfection. It's a skill that develops over time with consistent practice. Even if you can only manage to eat one meal a day mindfully at first, that's a significant step in the right direction. Gradually, you can work towards incorporating mindfulness into more of your eating experiences.

Slowing down during meals is another crucial aspect of mindful eating. In our busy lives, it's all too easy to rush through our food, barely tasting it as we wolf it down. However, this rapid eating not only robs us of the pleasure of our meals but can also lead to overeating. It takes approximately 20 minutes for our brains to register feelings of fullness, so when we eat too quickly, we may consume far more than we need before our body has a chance to signal that we're satisfied.

To combat this tendency, try setting down your utensils between bites. Take the time to chew your food thoroughly, aiming for 20 to 30 chews per mouthful. This not only slows down your eating but also aids in digestion and allows you to fully experience the flavors and textures of your food. You might be surprised at how much more satisfying your meals become when you give them your full attention and take the time to savor each bite.

Another effective strategy for slowing down is to engage in conversation during meals, particularly if you're dining with others. This natural pause between bites can help pace your eating and make the meal a more enjoyable social experience. However, be mindful that the conversation doesn't become so engrossing that you lose focus on your food entirely. Strive for a balance between social interaction and awareness of your eating.

As you become more adept at slowing down and savoring your meals, you'll likely find that you're more easily able to recognize your body's hunger and fullness cues. This awareness is a cornerstone of mindful eating and can be transformative in your relationship with food. Many of us have lost touch with these internal signals, either through years of restrictive dieting or habitual overeating. Reconnecting with these cues can help us eat in a way that truly nourishes our bodies.

Hunger, in its truest form, is a physical sensation. It might manifest as a gnawing feeling in your stomach, a slight headache, or a decrease in energy levels. It's important to distinguish this physical hunger from emotional hunger, which might be triggered by stress, boredom, or other feelings. Emotional hunger often comes on suddenly and craves specific comfort foods, whereas physical hunger develops more gradually and can be satisfied by a variety of foods.

Before you begin eating, take a moment to assess your hunger level. You might find it helpful to use a hunger scale, where 1 represents extreme hunger and 10 represents uncomfortably full. Ideally, you want to begin eating when you're at about a 3 or 4 on this scale – definitely hungry, but not ravenous. This helps prevent overeating that can occur when we wait until we're excessively hungry to have a meal.

As you eat, periodically check in with your body. How full do you feel? Are you still enjoying your food as much as you were at the beginning of the meal? The goal is to stop eating when you're comfortably satisfied, not stuffed. This point is often described as feeling about 80% full. It might take some practice to recognize this level of satiety, especially if you're used to eating until you feel very full. Be patient with yourself as you learn to interpret your body's signals.

Renowned eating psychologist and author Evelyn Tribole offers valuable insight on this topic: "Mindful eating is about awareness. When you eat mindfully, you slow down, pay attention to the food you're eating, and savor every bite." This simple yet profound statement encapsulates the essence of what we're striving for with this practice.

It's worth noting that recognizing fullness cues can be particularly challenging in our modern food environment, where we're often presented with large portions and encouraged to clean our plates. Remember that it's okay to leave food on your plate if you're feeling satisfied. You might find it helpful to use smaller plates or to serve yourself smaller portions initially, knowing you can always get more if you're still hungry.

As you embark on your mindful eating journey, you may encounter some common challenges. One of these is the urge to multitask during meals. In our busy lives, it can feel productive to catch up on work emails, scroll through social media, or watch TV while we eat. However, these distractions pull our attention away from our food and make it difficult to eat mindfully.

Try to create a dedicated eating environment free from these distractions. This might mean designating a specific place in your home for meals, away from your workspace or the TV. If you typically eat lunch at your desk, consider taking your meal to a nearby park or a break room instead. These small changes in your environment can make a big difference in your ability to focus on your food.

Another challenge you might face is dealing with time constraints. Many of us feel rushed during meals, whether due to busy work schedules or family obligations. While it's not always possible to have a leisurely meal, even taking an extra five minutes to eat more slowly can make a difference. You might find it helpful to schedule your meals and snacks, treating them as important appointments in your day rather than afterthoughts.

As you practice mindful eating, you may notice changes not only in how you eat but also in what you choose to eat. When we're fully present and attentive during meals, we're more likely to notice how different foods make us feel. You might find that certain foods leave you feeling energized and satisfied, while others leave you feeling sluggish or uncomfortably full. This awareness can naturally guide you towards making healthier food choices without the need for strict rules or deprivation.

Dr. Susan Albers, a clinical psychologist and expert in mindful eating, notes: "Mindful eating is not about being perfect, always eating the right things, or never allowing yourself to eat on-the-go again. It's about balance, choice and experience." This perspective underscores the flexibility and compassion inherent in the practice of mindful eating.

As we conclude this chapter on mindful eating, it's important to remember that this is just the beginning of your journey. Like any new habit, mindful eating takes time and practice to become second nature. Be patient with yourself as you learn and grow. Celebrate the small victories, like the first time you notice you're full before your plate is empty, or when you truly savor a meal without any distractions.

Remember, mindful eating is not about rigid rules or perfectionism. It's about developing a more conscious, intentional relationship with food. As you move forward, you'll find that this foundational habit supports and enhances all the other nutritional changes you'll be making. It sets the stage for a more balanced, satisfying approach to eating that can last a lifetime.

As we look ahead to the next chapter, we'll build on this foundation of mindfulness to explore another crucial aspect of healthy eating: portion control. We'll discover how to achieve satiety and nutritional balance without feeling deprived, using the awareness we've cultivated through mindful eating practices. This next step will further empower you to make sustainable, positive changes in your diet, one bite-sized habit at a time.

Chapter 7: Portion Control Without Deprivation

As we transition from the practice of mindful eating, we now turn our attention to another crucial aspect of developing healthy eating habits: portion control. While mindful eating helps us become more aware of our food and eating experiences, portion control allows us to manage the quantity of food we consume without feeling deprived. This chapter will explore practical strategies for managing portion sizes, helping you feel satisfied with less, and ultimately supporting your journey towards a healthier relationship with food.

Visual guides for portion sizes can be incredibly helpful in developing an intuitive sense of appropriate serving sizes. One of the most common visual guides is the "hand method." This technique uses different parts of your hand to estimate portion sizes for various food groups. For instance, a serving of protein, such as chicken or fish, should be about the size and thickness of your palm. A serving of carbohydrates, like rice or pasta, should fit in your cupped hand. Vegetables can be more generous, with a serving size equivalent to two open handfuls. For fats, such as oils or butter, limit the portion to the size of your fingertip or thumb.

Another useful visual guide is the "plate method." This approach involves dividing your plate into sections: half of the plate should be filled with non-starchy vegetables, one-quarter with lean protein, and one-quarter with complex carbohydrates. This simple visual representation can help you create balanced meals without the need for precise measurements or calorie counting. By consistently using these visual guides, you'll gradually internalize appropriate portion sizes, making it easier to maintain healthy eating habits even when dining out or in situations where measuring tools aren't available.

It's important to note that portion sizes have grown significantly over the past few decades, contributing to the obesity epidemic. Dr. Lisa Young, a renowned nutritionist and portion size expert, states in her book "The Portion Teller Plan": "Portion sizes have increased dramatically over the past 30 years, and there is overwhelming evidence linking growing portion sizes to the rise in obesity." This phenomenon, often referred to as "portion distortion," has led many people to consume far more calories than they need without realizing it. By becoming more aware of appropriate portion sizes and using visual guides, you can combat this trend and take control of your calorie intake.

Using smaller plates and bowls is a simple yet effective strategy for managing portion sizes. This approach leverages a psychological principle known as the Delboeuf illusion, which suggests that the size of a circle appears larger or smaller depending on the size of the circle surrounding it. In the context of eating, this means that the same amount of food will appear more substantial on a smaller plate than on a larger one. This visual trick can help you feel more satisfied with less food.

A study published in the Journal of Consumer Research found that participants who used smaller plates served themselves less food and consumed fewer calories overall. The researchers concluded that "the size of a food portion, when placed on a plate, appears larger when the plate is smaller rather than larger." By simply switching to smaller plates, you can create the illusion of a fuller plate while actually consuming less food.

Implementing this strategy doesn't require a complete overhaul of your dinnerware. Start by using salad plates instead of dinner plates for your main meals. For snacks and desserts, opt for small bowls or ramekins rather than larger serving dishes. Over time, you'll find that these smaller portions become the new normal, and you'll feel satisfied with less food.

It's worth noting that while smaller plates can be helpful, they're not a magic solution. It's still important to be mindful of what you're putting on your plate and to listen to your body's hunger and fullness cues. The goal is to use smaller plates as a tool to support your portion control efforts, not as a way to trick yourself into eating less than your body needs.

Strategies for feeling satisfied with less food are essential for successful portion control without deprivation. One key approach is to focus on nutrient-dense foods that provide a high level of satiety. Foods high in protein and fiber are particularly effective at promoting feelings of fullness. For example, including a source of lean protein like chicken, fish, or legumes in your meals can help you feel satisfied for longer periods. Similarly, high-fiber foods like vegetables, whole grains, and fruits can add volume to your meals without significantly increasing calorie content.

Another strategy is to practice the concept of volumetrics, developed by Dr. Barbara Rolls, a professor of nutritional sciences at Penn State University. This approach involves eating foods with a high water content, which adds volume to meals without adding calories. In her book "The Ultimate Volumetrics Diet," Dr. Rolls explains, "Water adds weight and volume to foods but not calories. Foods with a high water content have a lower energy density, meaning they have fewer calories per gram." By incorporating water-rich foods like soups, salads, and fruits into your meals, you can eat a larger volume of food while consuming fewer calories overall.

Eating slowly and mindfully, as discussed in the previous chapter, also plays a crucial role in feeling satisfied with less food. It takes about 20 minutes for your brain to register feelings of fullness. By slowing down your eating pace, you give your body time to recognize that it's becoming full, which can prevent overeating. Additionally, taking the time to savor your food and appreciate its flavors and textures can increase your overall satisfaction with the meal, making you less likely to want additional servings.

Incorporating appetite-regulating foods into your meals can also help manage portion sizes naturally. For instance, foods rich in omega-3 fatty acids, such as fatty fish, walnuts, and flaxseeds, have been shown to increase feelings of fullness. Similarly, foods with a low glycemic index, which cause a slower and more gradual rise in blood sugar levels, can help stabilize appetite and reduce cravings. Examples include whole grains, legumes, and most fruits and vegetables.

It's also important to address the psychological aspects of feeling satisfied with less food. Often, the desire to eat large portions is driven by emotional factors rather than genuine hunger. Learning to distinguish between physical hunger and emotional eating can be a powerful tool in managing portion sizes. Keep a food diary that includes not only what you eat but also your emotional state before and after eating. This can help you identify patterns and develop strategies to address emotional eating without relying on large portions of food.

Implementing these strategies for portion control without deprivation requires patience and consistency. It's normal to experience some initial resistance as your body and mind adjust to smaller portion sizes. However, with time and practice, you'll likely find that you feel just as satisfied—if not more so—with appropriately sized portions. Remember, the goal is not to restrict yourself, but to find a sustainable way of eating that nourishes your body and supports your overall health goals.

As you continue to work on portion control, it's important to maintain a flexible and compassionate approach. There will be times when you eat more than you intended, and that's okay. The key is to view these instances as learning opportunities rather than failures. Each meal is a chance to practice your portion control skills and refine your approach.

In the next chapter, we'll explore the often-overlooked aspect of nutrition: hydration. Proper hydration is not only essential for overall health but can also play a significant role in managing appetite and supporting your portion control efforts. We'll discuss the importance of adequate fluid intake and explore creative ways to increase your water consumption throughout the day.

Chapter 8: Hydration Habits

As we transition from our exploration of portion control, let's dive into an often overlooked yet crucial aspect of nutrition: hydration. The importance of proper hydration cannot be overstated, as it forms the foundation of every bodily function and plays a pivotal role in our overall health and well-being. In this chapter, we'll explore the significance of staying adequately hydrated, discover creative ways to increase water intake, and learn strategies for reducing sugary and caloric beverages.

Water is life. This simple statement encapsulates the profound importance of hydration in our daily lives. Every cell, tissue, and organ in our body depends on water to function optimally. From regulating body temperature and aiding digestion to supporting cognitive function and maintaining healthy skin, water is involved in countless physiological processes. Yet, despite its critical role, many people struggle to maintain proper hydration levels.

The human body is composed of approximately 60% water, with some organs, such as the brain and heart, containing even higher percentages. This high water content underscores the need for consistent replenishment. Dehydration, even in mild forms, can lead to a host of issues including fatigue, headaches, poor concentration, and decreased physical performance. In more severe cases, it can result in serious health complications.

One of the most common questions regarding hydration is, "How much water should I drink?" While the oft-cited recommendation of eight 8-ounce glasses (about 2 liters) per day is a good starting point, individual needs can vary based on factors such as age, sex, activity level, climate, and overall health. A more personalized approach is to listen to your body's thirst signals and observe the color of your urine. Pale yellow urine generally indicates adequate hydration, while dark yellow or amber-colored urine suggests you need to increase your fluid intake.

It's important to note that hydration isn't just about drinking plain water. While water should be your primary source of hydration, other beverages and even certain foods can contribute to your daily fluid intake. However, not all sources of hydration are created equal, and some can have negative health impacts if consumed in excess.

Let's explore some creative ways to increase your water intake. For many people, the taste (or lack thereof) of plain water can be a barrier to proper hydration. If this resonates with you, consider infusing your water with natural flavors. Adding slices of lemon, lime, or orange not only enhances the taste but also provides a boost of vitamin C. Cucumber, mint, or berries can create refreshing combinations that make drinking water more enjoyable. Herbal teas, both hot and iced, are another excellent way to increase fluid intake while enjoying a variety of flavors.

For those who struggle to remember to drink water throughout the day, technology can be a helpful ally. There are numerous smartphone apps designed to track water intake and send reminders. Some even gamify the experience, turning hydration into a fun challenge. Another simple yet effective strategy is to keep a water bottle visible and within reach at all times. Choose a bottle you enjoy using and consider marking it with time-based goals to encourage regular sipping throughout the day.

Eating water-rich foods is another clever way to boost your hydration levels. Fruits and vegetables with high water content, such as watermelon, cucumbers, tomatoes, and zucchini, can contribute significantly to your daily fluid intake. Not only do these foods help with hydration, but they also provide essential vitamins, minerals, and fiber.

While increasing water intake is crucial, it's equally important to reduce the consumption of sugary and caloric beverages. Many people unknowingly consume a significant portion of their daily calories through drinks. Sodas, energy drinks, and even fruit juices can be loaded with sugar and empty calories, contributing to weight gain and increasing the risk of chronic diseases like type 2 diabetes.

The transition away from sugary drinks can be challenging, especially if they've been a regular part of your diet. One effective strategy is to gradually dilute these beverages with water or seltzer water. Over time, you can increase the dilution until you've completely phased out the sugary drink. For those who enjoy carbonated beverages, sparkling water with a splash of 100% fruit juice can provide a satisfying alternative with far fewer calories and less sugar.

Coffee and tea, when consumed without added sugar or high-calorie creamers, can be part of a healthy hydration strategy. However, it's important to be mindful of their caffeine content, as excessive caffeine intake can have a mild diuretic effect. For most people, moderate consumption of caffeinated beverages doesn't significantly impact hydration levels, but it's best to balance them with plenty of water throughout the day.

Alcohol is another beverage category that requires careful consideration when it comes to hydration. Alcoholic drinks can have a dehydrating effect on the body, as alcohol acts as a diuretic, increasing urine production. If you choose to consume alcohol, it's wise to alternate each alcoholic drink with a glass of water. This not only helps counteract the dehydrating effects but can also slow down alcohol consumption, promoting more responsible drinking habits.

For those looking to make a significant impact on their health and hydration habits, consider implementing a "water first" policy. This means starting each day with a glass of water before consuming any other beverages or foods. Similarly, make it a habit to have a glass of water before each meal. Not only does this boost your hydration levels, but it can also help with portion control by creating a sense of fullness before eating.

It's worth noting that while increasing water intake is generally beneficial, there are situations where excessive water consumption can be harmful. Conditions such as congestive heart failure or certain kidney problems may require fluid restriction. Always consult with a healthcare professional if you have concerns about your hydration needs, especially if you have underlying health conditions.

As we cultivate better hydration habits, it's important to approach this change with patience and self-compassion. Like any other habit, consistent hydration takes time to become second nature.

Celebrate small victories, such as choosing water over a sugary drink or remembering to carry your water bottle to work. These small steps compound over time, leading to significant improvements in your overall health and well-being.

Remember, proper hydration is not just about quenching thirst; it's about nourishing your body at the most fundamental level. By prioritizing hydration and making conscious choices about the beverages you consume, you're laying the groundwork for better health, improved energy levels, and enhanced cognitive function.

As we conclude our exploration of hydration habits, consider how these strategies can integrate with the mindful eating practices and portion control techniques we've discussed in previous chapters. Each of these bite-sized habits works synergistically, creating a comprehensive approach to nutrition that goes beyond simply what we eat to encompass how we nourish and hydrate our bodies.

In the next chapter, we'll shift our focus to the first meal of the day, exploring how to start your mornings right with nutritious and satisfying breakfast options. We'll discover how a well-balanced morning meal can set the tone for a day of mindful, healthful eating, and learn strategies for overcoming common breakfast obstacles. Let's continue our journey towards transformative, sustainable dietary habits, one bite-sized change at a time.

Chapter 9: Breakfast: Starting Your Day Right

As we transition from our exploration of hydration habits, we now turn our attention to the first meal of the day, often hailed as the most important. Breakfast sets the tone for your entire day, influencing your energy levels, cognitive function, and even your food choices later on. In this chapter, we'll delve into the art of crafting a nutritious morning meal, explore quick and easy breakfast ideas, and tackle common obstacles that prevent many from enjoying this crucial meal.

The importance of a balanced breakfast cannot be overstated. As the word itself suggests, breakfast "breaks" the overnight "fast" our bodies undergo during sleep. During this fasting period, our bodies deplete their readily available energy stores, and breakfast replenishes these stores, kickstarting our metabolism for the day ahead. Dr. Daniela Jakubowicz, a professor at Tel Aviv University, explains, "Eating a high-calorie breakfast and a low-calorie dinner can help you lose weight and decrease your risk of metabolic syndrome."

A well-balanced breakfast provides your body with essential nutrients and energy to fuel your morning activities. It helps stabilize blood sugar levels, which is crucial for maintaining steady energy and focus throughout the day. Research published in the American Journal of Clinical Nutrition has shown that people who eat breakfast regularly tend to have better overall diet quality and are more likely to maintain a healthy weight compared to those who skip this meal.

However, despite its importance, breakfast is often the most neglected meal of the day. Many people cite lack of time, absence of appetite in the morning, or simply not knowing what to eat as reasons for skipping breakfast. These challenges are not insurmountable, and with the right strategies, anyone can incorporate a nutritious breakfast into their daily routine.

When considering what constitutes a balanced morning meal, it's essential to include a combination of complex carbohydrates, lean proteins, and healthy fats. Complex carbohydrates, such as whole grains, provide a steady release of energy throughout the morning. Protein helps to keep you feeling full and satisfied, reducing the likelihood of mid-morning snacking on less nutritious options. Healthy fats, like those found in avocados or nuts, contribute to satiety and aid in the absorption of fat-soluble vitamins.

One quick and nutritious breakfast idea is a bowl of steel-cut oats topped with fresh berries, a sprinkle of chopped nuts, and a dollop of Greek yogurt. This combination offers complex carbohydrates from the oats, antioxidants from the berries, healthy fats and additional protein from the nuts, and a protein boost from the Greek yogurt. Preparation can be streamlined by using overnight oats methods, where the oats are soaked in milk or a milk alternative overnight, ready to eat in the morning with minimal effort.

For those who prefer a savory start to the day, a whole grain toast topped with mashed avocado and a poached egg can be an excellent choice. The whole grain bread provides complex carbohydrates, the avocado offers healthy fats, and the egg delivers a high-quality protein source. This meal can be prepared in under 10 minutes, making it feasible even on busy mornings.

Smoothies are another fantastic option for a quick and nutritious breakfast, especially for those who struggle with appetite in the early hours. A smoothie made with spinach, banana, Greek yogurt, and a scoop of nut butter offers a balance of carbohydrates, proteins, and healthy fats, along with a hefty dose of vitamins and minerals. The beauty of smoothies lies in their versatility – ingredients can be easily swapped based on personal preferences or what's available in your kitchen.

For those who need an on-the-go option, preparing breakfast burritos in advance can be a game-changer. Whole wheat tortillas filled with scrambled eggs, black beans, diced vegetables, and a sprinkle of cheese can be wrapped and frozen. In the morning, simply reheat in the microwave for a portable, balanced meal. This method of batch preparation can save significant time during busy weekday mornings.

Despite these convenient options, many people still face obstacles when it comes to establishing a regular breakfast habit. One common challenge is a lack of appetite in the morning. This can often be addressed by gradually introducing small amounts of food earlier in the day. Start with something light, like a piece of fruit or a small yogurt, and slowly increase the quantity over time as your body adjusts to eating earlier.

Time constraints are another frequently cited barrier to eating breakfast. However, with proper planning and preparation, this obstacle can be overcome. Preparing components of your breakfast the night before, such as chopping fruits or portioning out dry ingredients, can significantly reduce morning prep time. Keeping a well-stocked pantry with easy breakfast items like whole grain cereals, nuts, and dried fruits can also make throwing together a quick meal much easier.

For those who find themselves rushing out the door without time for a sit-down meal, it's important to have grab-and-go options readily available. Hard-boiled eggs, whole fruit, and individually portioned containers of Greek yogurt or cottage cheese are all portable, nutrient-dense choices that require minimal preparation.

Another common breakfast pitfall is relying on convenience foods that are often high in sugar and low in nutritional value. Many popular breakfast cereals, pastries, and flavored yogurts fall into this category. While these may seem like quick and easy options, they often lead to energy crashes later in the morning and don't provide the sustained fuel your body needs. Instead, opt for whole, minimally processed foods whenever possible.

It's also worth noting that what constitutes a "breakfast food" is largely a cultural construct. There's no rule saying you can't have a bowl of vegetable soup or a leftover chicken breast for breakfast if that's what appeals to you. The key is to focus on balanced nutrition rather than adhering to traditional breakfast norms.

For those with more time on weekends, breakfast can be an opportunity for more elaborate meals and family bonding. Whole grain pancakes topped with fresh fruit, omelets filled with vegetables, or homemade granola paired with yogurt and honey are all delicious options that can make breakfast feel special.

These more involved meals can also be an opportunity to batch cook items for the week ahead, such as a large frittata that can be portioned and reheated on busy mornings.

As we conclude our exploration of breakfast habits, it's clear that this meal plays a crucial role in setting the stage for a day of balanced eating. By prioritizing a nutritious morning meal, you're not only fueling your body for immediate tasks but also laying the groundwork for better food choices throughout the day. Remember, the goal is progress, not perfection. Start with small changes, like committing to eating something nutritious within an hour of waking, and build from there.

As we move forward, we'll explore how to maintain this momentum of healthy eating throughout the day. In the next chapter, we'll dive into the world of smart snacking, learning how to choose nutrient-dense options that bridge the gap between meals and keep us energized throughout the day. The habits we form around breakfast set the tone for our entire day's eating patterns, making it a critical component of our overall nutrition strategy.

Chapter 10: Snacking Smartly

As we transition from our discussion on breakfast habits, it's important to recognize that our eating behaviors extend far beyond the morning meal. Snacking, often overlooked in traditional diet plans, plays a crucial role in our overall nutrition and can significantly impact our energy levels, mood, and even our main meal choices. In this chapter, we'll explore the art of snacking smartly, focusing on choosing nutrient-dense options, preparing healthy snacks in advance, and managing those pesky snack cravings.

Choosing nutrient-dense snacks

The key to smart snacking lies in selecting foods that pack a nutritional punch. Nutrient-dense snacks provide essential vitamins, minerals, and other beneficial compounds while typically being lower in calories compared to their less nutritious counterparts. These snacks not only satisfy hunger but also contribute to your overall health and well-being.

One excellent example of a nutrient-dense snack is a handful of raw nuts. Almonds, walnuts, and pistachios are rich in healthy fats, protein, and fiber, making them an ideal choice to keep you satiated between meals. A study published in the Journal of the American Heart Association found that consuming 1.5 ounces of almonds daily as a snack, instead of a high-carbohydrate muffin with equivalent calories, improved cardiovascular risk factors in adults with elevated LDL cholesterol.

Fresh fruits are another fantastic option for nutrient-dense snacking. Berries, for instance, are not only low in calories but also high in antioxidants, which help protect your cells from damage. A cup of mixed berries can provide a significant portion of your daily vitamin C requirement while satisfying your sweet tooth naturally. Pairing fruits with a source of protein or healthy fat, such as Greek yogurt or a small piece of cheese, can help balance blood sugar levels and keep you feeling full for longer.

Vegetables, often underutilized as snacks, offer a wealth of nutrients with minimal calories. Baby carrots, cherry tomatoes, and sliced bell peppers are convenient, crunchy options that can be enjoyed on their own or paired with hummus for added protein and healthy fats. The fiber content in vegetables aids digestion and promotes a feeling of fullness, making them an excellent choice for those looking to manage their weight without feeling deprived.

For those with a savory palate, hard-boiled eggs make an excellent snack choice. Packed with high-quality protein and essential nutrients like vitamin D and choline, eggs can help curb hunger and provide sustained energy. Research has shown that consuming eggs as a snack can lead to increased feelings of fullness and reduced calorie intake at subsequent meals.

When considering packaged snacks, it's crucial to read nutrition labels carefully. Look for options with minimal added sugars, hydrogenated oils, and artificial additives. Whole grain crackers with natural nut butter, unsweetened dried fruit, or air-popped popcorn can be good choices when you're on the go and need a shelf-stable option.

It's worth noting that even nutrient-dense snacks should be consumed in moderation. Portion control remains important, as overconsumption of any food, no matter how healthy, can lead to weight gain and nutritional imbalances. Use small containers or pre-portion your snacks to avoid mindless overeating.

Preparing healthy snacks in advance

One of the biggest challenges in maintaining healthy snacking habits is convenience. When hunger strikes, it's all too easy to reach for whatever is readily available, which often means processed, high-calorie options. This is where preparation becomes your greatest ally in the quest for smarter snacking.

Dedicating time each week to snack preparation can dramatically improve your eating habits. This practice, often referred to as "meal prepping," isn't just for main meals – it's equally beneficial for snacks. By having nutritious options readily available, you're setting yourself up for success and making it easier to resist less healthy alternatives.

Start by washing and cutting fresh fruits and vegetables as soon as you bring them home from the grocery store. Store them in clear containers at eye level in your refrigerator. This visibility serves as a visual cue, making you more likely to choose these healthy options when you open the fridge door. Pre-cut veggies can be paired with individual portions of hummus or guacamole, creating a grab-and-go snack that requires no additional preparation.

Homemade trail mix is another excellent option for advance preparation. Combine raw nuts, seeds, and a small amount of dried fruit for a balanced mix of protein, healthy fats, and natural sugars. Portion these into small containers or bags for easy grabbing throughout the week. This approach not only ensures you have a healthy snack on hand but also helps with portion control.

Greek yogurt parfaits can be prepared in advance and stored in the refrigerator for several days. Layer Greek yogurt with fresh berries and a sprinkle of low-sugar granola for a snack that's both satisfying and nutritious. The protein in the yogurt helps keep you full, while the fruit provides essential vitamins and antioxidants.

For those who enjoy baking, preparing a batch of healthy muffins or energy balls at the beginning of the week can provide a week's worth of nutritious snacks. Opt for recipes that use whole grain flours, natural sweeteners like mashed bananas or dates, and include ingredients like chia seeds or ground flaxseed for added nutrition. These homemade treats can be individually wrapped and frozen, allowing you to defrost only what you need each day.

Hard-boiled eggs are another excellent snack that can be prepared in advance. Boil a dozen eggs at the start of the week, peel them, and store them in the refrigerator. They'll stay fresh for up to seven days, providing a quick protein boost whenever you need it.

When preparing snacks in advance, it's important to consider food safety. Always store perishable items in the refrigerator and be mindful of expiration dates. Use airtight containers to keep foods fresh and prevent cross-contamination.

By investing time in snack preparation, you're not only ensuring that you have healthy options available but also saving time and reducing stress during busy weekdays. This proactive approach to snacking can help you maintain consistent energy levels throughout the day and support your overall nutrition goals.

Managing snack cravings

Even with the best preparation and intentions, managing snack cravings can be challenging. Cravings are complex phenomena influenced by various factors including hormones, emotions, habits, and even our environment. Understanding these triggers and developing strategies to manage them is crucial for maintaining healthy snacking habits.

One effective approach to managing cravings is to practice mindful eating. This involves paying full attention to the experience of eating and drinking, both inside and outside the body. When you feel a craving coming on, pause and ask yourself if you're truly hungry or if something else is driving the desire to eat. Are you bored, stressed, or simply responding to an environmental cue like seeing a food advertisement?

If you determine that you're experiencing true hunger, reach for one of your prepared healthy snacks. If, however, you realize that your craving is emotionally driven, try engaging in an alternative activity. This could be taking a short walk, practicing deep breathing exercises, or calling a friend. Often, the craving will pass once you've redirected your attention.

It's also important to recognize that completely restricting yourself from foods you crave can sometimes backfire, leading to eventual overindulgence. Instead, practice moderation and planned indulgence. Allow yourself small portions of treats occasionally, savoring them fully without guilt. This approach can help prevent feelings of deprivation that might lead to binge eating later.

Staying hydrated can also help manage snack cravings. Sometimes, what we perceive as hunger is actually thirst. Make it a habit to drink a glass of water when you feel a craving coming on. If you're still hungry after 15-20 minutes, then reach for a nutritious snack.

Balancing your meals throughout the day can also help reduce snack cravings. Ensure that your main meals include a good balance of protein, complex carbohydrates, and healthy fats. This combination helps stabilize blood sugar levels and keeps you feeling satisfied for longer periods.

For those who find themselves craving specific types of foods, it can be helpful to analyze the potential nutritional deficiencies that might be driving these cravings. For instance, chocolate cravings might indicate a need for magnesium, which can be addressed by incorporating more magnesium-rich foods like spinach, pumpkin seeds, or black beans into your diet.

It's also worth examining your sleep habits when dealing with persistent snack cravings. Lack of sleep can disrupt hormones that regulate hunger and fullness, potentially leading to increased cravings and overeating. Prioritizing good sleep hygiene can have a positive impact on your eating habits during the day.

Stress management is another crucial aspect of controlling snack cravings. Chronic stress can lead to emotional eating and cravings for high-calorie, comfort foods. Incorporating stress-reduction techniques such as meditation, yoga, or regular exercise into your routine can help mitigate stress-induced cravings.

Remember that changing ingrained habits takes time and patience. If you find yourself giving in to unhealthy snacking occasionally, don't view it as a failure. Instead, use it as a learning opportunity. Reflect on what led to the choice and how you can prepare differently in the future. Cultivating self-compassion and viewing your health journey as a long-term process rather than a series of "good" or "bad" choices can help you maintain a positive mindset and stay motivated.

As we conclude our exploration of smart snacking strategies, it's clear that this aspect of our diet plays a significant role in our overall nutrition and well-being. By choosing nutrient-dense options, preparing snacks in advance, and developing effective strategies to manage cravings, you're equipping yourself with powerful tools to support your health goals. These bite-sized habits, when consistently applied, can lead to substantial improvements in your diet and overall health.

As we move forward, we'll turn our attention to another crucial aspect of daily nutrition – lunch on the go. In the next chapter, we'll explore how to maintain healthy eating habits even when faced with the challenges of a busy lifestyle and limited time for meal preparation.

Chapter 11: Lunch on the Go

As we transition from our morning routines and the breakfast habits we've cultivated, we find ourselves facing the midday challenge: lunch. For many, this meal presents a unique set of obstacles, particularly when juggling busy professional lives or hectic schedules. The importance of a nutritious lunch cannot be overstated, as it provides the fuel needed to power through the afternoon and can significantly impact our overall dietary health. In this chapter, we'll explore strategies to ensure that your midday meal aligns with your nutritional goals, even when time is at a premium.

Meal prep strategies for busy professionals have become increasingly popular, and for good reason. The concept of preparing meals in advance is not new, but its application to modern lifestyles has revolutionized how we approach lunch. By dedicating a small portion of your weekend or evening to meal preparation, you can set yourself up for a week of healthful, convenient lunches that require minimal effort during busy workdays.

One effective approach is the 'batch cooking' method. This involves preparing larger quantities of key ingredients that can be mixed and matched throughout the week. For instance, you might grill several chicken breasts, roast a variety of vegetables, and cook a large batch of quinoa or brown rice. These components can then be combined in different ways to create diverse lunches throughout the week, preventing the monotony that often leads to unhealthy food choices.

Another strategy is the 'assembly line' approach to meal prep. Set up containers and fill each with a portion of protein, complex carbohydrates, and vegetables. This method allows for quick grab-and-go lunches that are balanced and satisfying. Remember, the key to successful meal prep is variety. As nutrition expert Dr. Marion Nestle points out, "Variety is not only the spice of life; it's the key to nutritional adequacy." By including a range of colorful vegetables, lean proteins, and whole grains, you ensure a broad spectrum of nutrients in your midday meals.

For those days when meal prep isn't possible or you find yourself without a packed lunch, navigating restaurant menus becomes an essential skill. The modern workplace often involves business lunches or quick bites between meetings, making it crucial to develop strategies for making healthful choices when eating out.

When faced with a restaurant menu, start by looking for keywords that indicate healthier preparation methods. Terms like 'grilled,' 'baked,' 'steamed,' or 'roasted' generally signify dishes that are lower in added fats compared to 'fried,' 'crispy,' or 'battered' options. Don't hesitate to ask your server about preparation methods or request modifications to make a dish healthier. Many restaurants are accustomed to accommodating dietary preferences and restrictions.

It's also wise to be mindful of portion sizes when dining out. Restaurant portions are often much larger than what we need for a single meal. Consider sharing a dish with a colleague or asking for a to-go container at the beginning of the meal to set aside half for later. This not only helps with portion control but also provides you with another meal, saving both money and time.

Salads can be an excellent choice for a restaurant lunch, but be cautious of high-calorie dressings and toppings. Request dressing on the side so you can control the amount used, and be mindful of additions like croutons, cheese, and nuts, which can quickly turn a light salad into a calorie-dense meal. Instead, look for salads that feature a variety of vegetables and lean proteins like grilled chicken or fish.

When it comes to beverages, water should be your go-to choice. Not only is it calorie-free, but proper hydration can also help you feel more satisfied with your meal. If you're craving something with more flavor, unsweetened iced tea or sparkling water with a slice of lemon can be refreshing alternatives to sugary sodas or high-calorie coffee drinks.

For those who prefer to bring lunch from home, balanced packed lunch ideas are essential. The key is to think beyond the traditional sandwich and chips. While sandwiches can be a convenient option, they often lack the variety and nutrient density needed for an optimal lunch. Instead, consider alternatives that incorporate a wider range of food groups and textures.

One popular option is the 'bento box' style lunch. This Japanese-inspired approach involves packing several small portions of different foods in a compartmentalized container. A typical bento might include a small portion of lean protein (such as grilled chicken or tofu), a serving of whole grains or starchy vegetables, an assortment of fresh vegetables, and a piece of fruit. This style of lunch not only ensures a balance of nutrients but also provides visual appeal and variety, making your midday meal more satisfying.

Grain-based salads are another excellent option for packed lunches. These can be prepared in advance and often taste even better after the flavors have had time to meld. A base of quinoa, farro, or brown rice can be combined with a variety of vegetables, nuts or seeds for crunch, and a lean protein source. Dress the salad lightly with a vinaigrette made from olive oil and vinegar or lemon juice, which will help keep the ingredients fresh and flavorful without becoming soggy.

Soups and stews can also make for hearty and nutritious packed lunches, especially in cooler months. Prepare a large batch at the beginning of the week and portion it out into individual containers. Pair your soup with a side of whole grain crackers or a small salad for a complete meal. As an added benefit, the act of eating soup can help you feel more satisfied due to its high water content and the time it takes to consume.

Don't forget the power of leftovers. Intentionally cooking extra portions at dinner can provide the basis for the next day's lunch. This not only saves time but also reduces food waste. Simply package the leftovers in a microwave-safe container for easy reheating at work.

When packing your lunch, consider investing in quality containers that are both leak-proof and microwave-safe. This will give you more flexibility in the types of foods you can bring and how you can reheat them. Additionally, include an ice pack or frozen water bottle to keep perishable items at a safe temperature until lunchtime.

Remember, the goal of these lunch strategies is not just to fill your stomach, but to provide your body with the nutrients it needs to function optimally throughout the afternoon. A well-balanced lunch can help prevent the dreaded mid-afternoon energy slump, keeping you focused and productive for the rest of the workday.

As we conclude our exploration of lunch strategies, it's important to remember that these habits, like all the bite-sized changes we've discussed, take time to develop. Be patient with yourself as you experiment with different meal prep techniques, restaurant ordering strategies, and packed lunch ideas. The key is to find approaches that work for your lifestyle and preferences while supporting your overall nutrition goals.

As we move forward, we'll turn our attention to the final meal of the day. Dinner presents its own set of challenges and opportunities, and in the next chapter, we'll explore how to create nutritious, satisfying evening meals that complement the healthy habits you're building throughout the day. Whether you're cooking for yourself, your family, or entertaining guests, the strategies we'll discuss will help you end your day on a nutritious note, setting the stage for restful sleep and another day of mindful eating.

CHAPTER 12: DINNER DONE RIGHT

As we transition from the challenges of lunch on the go, we now turn our attention to the final main meal of the day: dinner. This pivotal meal offers a unique opportunity to nourish our bodies, connect with loved ones, and wind down from the day's activities. However, for many, dinner can become a source of stress or a time when healthy eating habits falter. In this chapter, we'll explore strategies to make dinner a consistent, nutritious, and enjoyable part of your day.

Family-friendly, nutritious dinner recipes are the cornerstone of a successful evening meal routine. The key is to find a balance between dishes that appeal to various palates while ensuring they provide the necessary nutrients. One approach is to reimagine classic favorites with a healthier twist. For instance, a traditional spaghetti bolognese can be transformed by using whole grain pasta, lean ground turkey instead of beef, and incorporating a variety of vegetables into the sauce. This not only boosts the nutritional profile but also introduces children to a wider range of flavors and textures.

Another family-friendly option is the build-your-own bowl concept. Start with a base of brown rice, quinoa, or mixed greens. Offer a selection of lean proteins such as grilled chicken, baked tofu, or beans. Then, provide an array of colorful vegetables, both raw and cooked. Finally, include healthy fat options like avocado slices or a sprinkle of nuts. This approach allows each family member to customize their meal while ensuring a balanced plate.

It's also an excellent way to use up leftover vegetables and proteins from previous meals.

For those nights when time is particularly tight, having a repertoire of quick, nutritious recipes is invaluable. One-pan meals are excellent for these situations. A sheet pan dinner of roasted salmon with asparagus and sweet potato wedges, for example, can be prepared in under 30 minutes with minimal clean-up. Similarly, a stir-fry of mixed vegetables with tofu or lean meat over brown rice can be whipped up quickly and provides a balanced meal with protein, complex carbohydrates, and fiber.

It's worth noting that nutritious doesn't have to mean complicated. As nutrition expert Michael Pollan famously said, "Eat food. Not too much. Mostly plants." This simple philosophy can guide your dinner choices. A dinner of a baked sweet potato topped with black beans, salsa, and a dollop of Greek yogurt, served alongside a simple green salad, meets these criteria and can be prepared with minimal effort.

Batch cooking for convenience is another strategy that can revolutionize your dinner routine. This approach involves preparing larger quantities of food components that can be mixed and matched throughout the week. For instance, on a Sunday afternoon, you might roast a large pan of mixed vegetables, cook a pot of brown rice or quinoa, prepare a batch of grilled chicken breasts, and make a large salad. These components can then be combined in various ways throughout the week to create different meals.

One night, you might have a grain bowl with roasted vegetables and chicken. The next, you could use the same ingredients to make a wrap or a salad. This not only saves time during busy weeknights but also ensures that you always have nutritious options on hand, reducing the temptation to order takeout or rely on processed convenience foods.

When batch cooking, it's important to consider food safety.

Cooked foods should be cooled quickly and stored in the refrigerator within two hours of cooking. Most cooked dishes will keep in the refrigerator for 3-4 days, while raw vegetables typically last about a week. If you've prepared more than you can use within this timeframe, consider freezing portions for future use.

Another aspect of batch cooking is the preparation of complete meals that can be frozen and reheated later. Soups, stews, casseroles, and chili are excellent candidates for this approach. These meals can be a lifesaver on particularly hectic evenings or when you're too tired to cook. Having a stash of homemade, nutritious frozen meals can help you resist the allure of less healthy frozen dinner options.

Strategies for avoiding late-night overeating are crucial for maintaining a healthy eating pattern. Late-night eating, particularly of high-calorie, nutrient-poor foods, can disrupt sleep patterns and contribute to weight gain. One effective strategy is to establish a "kitchen closing time" after dinner. This mental cue can help reduce mindless snacking in the evening hours.

If you find yourself consistently hungry in the late evening, it might be a sign that your dinner isn't providing enough sustenance. Experiment with increasing the protein and fiber content of your evening meal. These nutrients promote feelings of fullness and can help curb late-night cravings. For instance, adding a serving of lentils to your dinner or including a side of roasted chickpeas can boost both protein and fiber intake.

Another strategy is to plan for a small, nutrient-dense evening snack if needed. This could be a small handful of nuts, a piece of fruit with a tablespoon of nut butter, or a small serving of Greek yogurt with berries. By planning this snack, you're less likely to reach for less healthy options out of sudden hunger or habit.

Hydration also plays a role in managing late-night eating. Sometimes, thirst can be mistaken for hunger. Make it a habit to drink a glass of water after dinner and keep a water bottle nearby in the evening. Herbal teas can also be a satisfying, calorie-free option that can help curb the urge to eat when you're not truly hungry.

Mindful eating practices are particularly important at dinner time. With the day's stresses and distractions, it's easy to fall into the habit of eating while watching television or scrolling through your phone. However, this distracted eating can lead to overconsumption and reduced satisfaction from your meal. Make an effort to eat dinner at a table, free from screens. Focus on the flavors, textures, and aromas of your food. This mindful approach can help you feel more satisfied with your meal and reduce the likelihood of unnecessary snacking later in the evening.

For families, dinner time presents an opportunity for connection and modeling healthy eating behaviors. Research has consistently shown that regular family meals are associated with better nutritional intake and lower risk of obesity in children and adolescents. Even if you can't manage a family dinner every night, aim for a few nights a week where everyone sits down together.

Use this time not just for eating, but for conversation and connection. Avoid discussions about contentious topics or disciplinary issues at the dinner table. Instead, focus on positive interactions. You might institute a practice where each family member shares something they're grateful for or a highlight from their day. This not only fosters a positive atmosphere but also slows down the pace of the meal, allowing for better digestion and recognition of fullness cues.

For those living alone, dinner time can still be an opportunity for mindful eating and self-care. Consider setting the table nicely, even if it's just for yourself. Use proper plates and utensils rather than eating out of containers. You might enjoy your meal while listening to relaxing music or an interesting podcast. The key is to make dinner a intentional, enjoyable experience rather than a rushed afterthought.

As we wrap up our discussion on mastering the dinner meal, it's important to remember that perfection is not the goal. There will be nights when takeout is the best option, or when a simple sandwich is all you have the energy to prepare. The key is to have strategies and habits in place that make nutritious dinners the norm rather than the exception.

In the next chapter, we'll explore how to tie all these individual meal strategies together through effective meal planning. We'll discuss how a little forethought and organization can make healthy eating easier and more consistent throughout the week. By mastering the art of meal planning, you'll be better equipped to navigate the challenges of busy schedules while still prioritizing your nutritional needs.

Chapter 13: Mastering Meal Planning

As we transition from our exploration of dinner strategies, we now turn our attention to a crucial aspect of maintaining healthy eating habits: meal planning. This chapter will delve into the art and science of creating a flexible meal plan, shopping with intention, and leveraging technology to streamline your meal planning process.

Creating a flexible meal plan is the cornerstone of successful long-term dietary changes. It's not about rigid schedules or monotonous repetition, but rather about crafting a framework that adapts to your lifestyle while supporting your nutritional goals. Begin by considering your weekly routine. Are there days when you're particularly busy and need quick, easy meals? Or times when you have more leisure to prepare elaborate dishes? Understanding your schedule is the first step in creating a plan that works for you.

Start by planning for a week at a time. This timeframe is long enough to provide variety and take advantage of batch cooking, yet short enough to remain manageable. Choose a consistent day each week to sit down and plan your meals. Many find Sunday evenings work well, allowing them to prepare for the week ahead. As you plan, consider incorporating leftovers into your schedule. For instance, if you're making a large batch of chili on Monday, plan to use it for lunch on Wednesday. This approach not only saves time but also reduces food waste.

Variety is key to maintaining interest in your meal plan. Aim to include different protein sources, grains, and vegetables throughout the week. This not only ensures a broad spectrum of nutrients but also keeps your palate engaged. Consider themes to make planning easier – perhaps Meatless Monday, Taco Tuesday, or Stir-Fry Friday. These themes provide structure while still allowing for creativity within each category.

Flexibility is crucial for long-term success. Life is unpredictable, and your meal plan should be able to accommodate unexpected changes. Perhaps you have a last-minute dinner invitation or a late meeting at work. Build in a few 'flex meals' each week – simple, quick options that you can fall back on when plans change. These might include a vegetable omelet, a hearty salad, or a grain bowl with pre-cooked components.

Once you have your meal plan in place, the next step is grocery shopping with intention. This is where many people falter, succumbing to impulse purchases or forgetting key ingredients. The key is to approach shopping as a strategic mission rather than a casual errand. Start by taking inventory of what you already have in your pantry, refrigerator, and freezer. This prevents unnecessary purchases and helps you use up items before they spoil.

Based on your meal plan and inventory, create a comprehensive shopping list. Organize this list by store sections (produce, dairy, meats, etc.) to make your trip more efficient. As nutrition expert Marion Nestle advises, "Shop the perimeter of the store where fresh foods are usually located." This strategy naturally steers you towards whole, unprocessed foods that form the basis of a healthy diet.

When shopping, stick to your list as much as possible. This doesn't mean you can't be flexible if you spot a great deal on a healthy item, but it does mean avoiding the temptation of processed snacks or unnecessary purchases. Pay attention to sales and seasonal produce, which can help you save money while ensuring you're getting the freshest ingredients.

Consider buying in bulk for non-perishable items and foods you use frequently. This can be more cost-effective and reduces the need for frequent shopping trips. However, be cautious not to overbuy perishables, as this can lead to food waste. Remember, the goal is to buy what you need for your planned meals, not to stock up unnecessarily.

In today's digital age, technology can be a powerful ally in streamlining your meal planning process. Numerous apps and websites are available to help you plan meals, generate shopping lists, and even order groceries online. These tools can save time and make the process more efficient and enjoyable.

Meal planning apps like Mealime, Plan to Eat, or Paprika allow you to input recipes, generate shopping lists, and even scale recipes based on the number of servings you need. Some apps also provide nutritional information, helping you ensure your meals are balanced and aligned with your health goals.

For grocery shopping, apps like AnyList or OurGroceries allow you to create and share lists, making it easy to collaborate with family members. Many of these apps also integrate with voice assistants, so you can add items to your list hands-free while cooking or when you notice you're running low on something.

Online grocery ordering and delivery services have become increasingly popular and can be a significant time-saver. Whether you choose curbside pickup or home delivery, these services allow you to stick to your list more easily, avoiding impulse purchases and saving time. However, be mindful of any additional fees and make sure to check the quality of produce and expiration dates when your order arrives.

Recipe websites and databases can be invaluable resources for meal planning. Sites like Epicurious, AllRecipes, or Yummly offer vast collections of recipes with user ratings and reviews. Many allow you to save recipes to your personal collection or meal plan. When exploring these resources, look for recipes that align with your nutritional goals and cooking skill level. Don't be afraid to modify recipes to suit your tastes or dietary needs.

While technology can be incredibly helpful, it's important not to become overly reliant on it. The most effective meal planning systems often combine digital tools with good old-fashioned pen and paper. Many people find that physically writing out their meal plan or shopping list helps cement it in their memory and makes them more likely to stick to it.

As you become more adept at meal planning, you'll likely develop your own system that works best for you. Some people prefer to plan every meal and snack, while others focus on dinners and leave other meals more flexible. You might find that planning for two weeks at a time works better for your schedule, or that you prefer to shop twice a week for the freshest produce.

Remember that meal planning is a skill that improves with practice. Don't be discouraged if your first attempts aren't perfect. Each week, take a few moments to reflect on what worked well and what could be improved. Perhaps you overestimated how much food you needed, or underestimated how long a particular recipe would take to prepare. Use these insights to refine your approach for the following week.

Meal planning can also be a wonderful opportunity to involve family members or housemates in the process of creating healthy eating habits. Encourage input on meal ideas, delegate shopping or cooking tasks, and use meal planning as a way to teach children about nutrition and cooking skills. This collaborative approach not only shares the workload but also increases buy-in from everyone involved, making it more likely that the plan will be followed.

As we conclude this chapter on mastering meal planning, it's clear that this skill is about much more than deciding what to eat. It's a powerful tool for taking control of your nutrition, reducing stress around food choices, and creating a sustainable approach to healthy eating. By creating a flexible plan, shopping with intention, and leveraging technology, you're setting yourself up for success in your journey towards better nutrition.

As we move forward, we'll explore how to navigate the challenges of social eating and special occasions while maintaining your commitment to healthy habits. These situations can often derail even the best-laid plans, but with the right strategies, you can enjoy social events without compromising your nutritional goals.

Chapter 14: Navigating Social Eating and Special Occasions

As we transition from the structured environment of meal planning discussed in the previous chapter, we now venture into the more unpredictable realm of social eating and special occasions. This aspect of our dietary journey often presents unique challenges that can test our commitment to healthy eating habits. However, with the right strategies and mindset, it's possible to maintain a balanced approach while still enjoying the social aspects of food.

Social eating is an integral part of human culture, fostering connections and creating shared experiences. From casual dinners with friends to elaborate holiday feasts, these occasions are often centered around food. The challenge lies in balancing our nutritional goals with the desire to participate fully in these social experiences. It's crucial to remember that healthy eating is not about deprivation or isolation, but rather about making informed choices that align with our overall well-being.

When it comes to eating out with friends, preparation is key. Many people find themselves anxious about restaurant meals, fearing they'll derail their healthy eating habits. However, with a bit of forethought, dining out can be both enjoyable and nutritious. One effective strategy is to review the menu in advance. Most restaurants now have their menus available online, allowing you to plan your meal before you even arrive. Look for options that include lean proteins, vegetables, and whole grains. Don't be afraid to ask for modifications – many establishments are happy to accommodate requests for dressings on the side, grilled instead of fried preparations, or extra vegetables in place of high-carb sides.

Another useful tactic when eating out is to practice mindful eating. This approach, which we explored in depth earlier in the book, is particularly valuable in social settings. Take the time to savor each bite, engaging in conversation between mouthfuls. This not only enhances your enjoyment of the meal but also helps you eat more slowly, allowing your body to register fullness before you overeat. Remember, it's not just about what you eat, but how you eat it.

Portion control can be particularly challenging when dining out, as restaurant servings are often much larger than what we need. One way to manage this is to ask for a to-go container at the beginning of the meal and immediately set aside half of your entree. This not only helps you avoid overeating but also provides you with a ready-made meal for the next day. Alternatively, consider sharing a main course with a friend and ordering an extra side of vegetables. This approach allows you to sample different dishes while keeping portions in check.

When it comes to alcohol consumption in social settings, moderation is key. Alcoholic beverages are often high in calories and can lower our inhibitions, leading to poor food choices. If you choose to drink, alternate alcoholic beverages with water or seltzer. This helps you stay hydrated and reduces overall calorie intake. Opt for drinks with lower calorie content, such as a glass of wine or a spirit with a calorie-free mixer, rather than sugary cocktails.

Holiday meals and celebrations present their own set of challenges. These occasions are often laden with emotional significance and family traditions, many of which revolve around food. It's important to approach these situations with a balanced mindset. Remember, a single meal or day of indulgence will not undo all your hard work. The key is to enjoy these special occasions without letting them derail your overall healthy eating habits.

One effective strategy for navigating holiday meals is to contribute a healthy dish to the gathering. This ensures that there's at least one option that aligns with your nutritional goals. It's also an opportunity to share delicious, nutritious recipes with friends and family, potentially inspiring others to incorporate healthier choices into their own diets.

During holiday meals, focus on filling your plate with a variety of foods, including plenty of vegetables and lean proteins. This doesn't mean you can't enjoy traditional holiday dishes – rather, it's about finding a balance. Take small portions of rich, indulgent foods, savoring them fully. This approach allows you to participate in the celebratory aspect of the meal without overindulging.

It's also important to be mindful of the non-food aspects of holiday gatherings. Engage in conversations, participate in activities, and focus on creating memories with loved ones. By shifting some of the emphasis away from food, you can fully enjoy the spirit of the occasion without feeling like you're missing out or restricted.

The concept of balance is crucial when it comes to indulgence and moderation. It's unrealistic and often counterproductive to completely abstain from treats or rich foods, especially during social occasions or celebrations. The key is to find a middle ground that allows for enjoyment without compromising your overall health goals.

One helpful approach is the 80/20 rule. This guideline suggests that if you make nutritious choices 80% of the time, you have some flexibility with the remaining 20%. This balance allows for the occasional indulgence without derailing your progress. It's important to note that this doesn't mean going overboard 20% of the time, but rather allowing yourself to enjoy less nutritious foods in moderation.

When you do indulge, do so mindfully and without guilt. Savor each bite, truly enjoying the experience. Pay attention to your body's signals of fullness and satisfaction. Often, a small portion of a favorite treat can be just as satisfying as a large amount, especially when eaten with full awareness and appreciation.

Remember, the goal of adopting healthy eating habits is not to achieve perfection, but to create a sustainable, enjoyable way of nourishing your body. Social eating and special occasions are part of a balanced, fulfilling life. By approaching these situations with mindfulness and preparation, you can navigate them successfully while staying true to your health goals.

Developing strategies for social eating situations is an ongoing process. What works for one person may not work for another, and what's effective in one situation might not be in another. Be patient with yourself as you learn to navigate these challenges. Each social eating experience is an opportunity to refine your approach and strengthen your commitment to your health journey.

As we conclude this chapter on navigating social eating and special occasions, it's important to reflect on how these strategies fit into your overall approach to nutrition. Remember, the bite-sized habits we've been cultivating throughout this book are designed to be flexible and adaptable to various life situations. In the next chapter, we'll explore how to overcome obstacles and setbacks in your healthy eating journey, providing you with tools to maintain your progress even when faced with challenges.

CHAPTER 15: OVERCOMING OBSTACLES AND SETBACKS

The path to healthier eating habits is rarely a straight line. As we embark on our journey to transform our diet one meal at a time, we inevitably encounter obstacles and experience setbacks. These challenges are not signs of failure, but rather opportunities for growth and learning. In this chapter, we'll explore strategies for dealing with common hurdles such as food cravings and emotional eating, techniques for getting back on track after slip-ups, and methods for building resilience in your healthy eating journey.

Dealing with food cravings is often one of the most significant challenges people face when trying to improve their eating habits. Cravings can be intense and seemingly uncontrollable, leading many to abandon their nutritional goals in moments of weakness. However, understanding the nature of cravings can help us develop effective strategies to manage them. Dr. Susan Peirce Thompson, a neuroscientist specializing in the psychology of eating, explains, "Cravings are not a sign of weakness or lack of willpower. They are a normal biological response to certain triggers in our environment or internal states."

One effective approach to managing cravings is to practice

mindful awareness. When a craving strikes, take a moment to pause and observe the sensation without judgment. Notice where you feel the craving in your body and what thoughts or emotions accompany it. This simple act of observation can create a space between the craving and your response, allowing you to make a more conscious choice about how to proceed.

Another strategy is to identify and address the underlying needs that may be driving your cravings. Often, cravings are not actually about the food itself but about a deeper emotional or physical need. For example, a craving for sweet foods might be your body's way of seeking comfort or energy. By recognizing these underlying needs, you can explore alternative ways to meet them that don't involve unhealthy eating.

Emotional eating is closely related to cravings and presents its own set of challenges. Many of us turn to food as a way to cope with stress, sadness, boredom, or other emotions. While this may provide temporary relief, it often leads to feelings of guilt and can derail our healthy eating efforts. Dr. Jane Ogden, a professor of health psychology, notes, "Emotional eating is a learned behavior that can be unlearned with practice and patience."

To address emotional eating, it's crucial to develop a toolkit of alternative coping strategies. This might include activities like going for a walk, practicing deep breathing exercises, calling a friend, or engaging in a hobby you enjoy. The key is to find healthy ways to process and express your emotions that don't involve food. It's also important to cultivate emotional awareness, learning to distinguish between physical hunger and emotional hunger.

Despite our best efforts, slip-ups are an inevitable part of any behavior change process. The key to long-term success is not to avoid slip-ups entirely, but to develop strategies for getting back on track quickly when they do occur. One powerful approach is to practice self-compassion. Dr. Kristin Neff, a leading researcher on self-compassion, explains, "Self-compassion involves treating yourself with the same kindness and understanding that you would offer a good friend. It's about recognizing that imperfection is part of the shared human experience."

When you experience a setback in your healthy eating journey, resist the urge to engage in harsh self-criticism. Instead, acknowledge the slip-up with kindness and curiosity. Ask yourself what you can learn from the experience and how you can use that knowledge to support your goals moving forward. Remember that one unhealthy meal or even one unhealthy day does not negate all of your progress. The most important thing is to return to your healthy habits as soon as possible, without allowing a temporary setback to turn into a prolonged deviation from your goals.

Building resilience is crucial for maintaining healthy eating habits over the long term. Resilience in this context refers to your ability to adapt to challenges and bounce back from setbacks. One way to build resilience is to focus on your "why" – the deeper reasons behind your desire to eat healthier. Perhaps you want to have more energy to play with your children, or you're motivated by a family history of health issues. Regularly connecting with these core motivations can help you stay committed to your goals even when faced with obstacles.

Another key aspect of resilience is developing a growth mindset about your eating habits. This means viewing challenges as opportunities for learning and growth rather than as failures. Dr. Carol Dweck, a psychologist known for her work on mindset, suggests, "In a growth mindset, challenges are exciting rather than threatening. So rather than thinking, oh, I'm going to reveal my weaknesses, you say, wow, here's a chance to grow."

Practicing flexibility in your approach to healthy eating can also enhance your resilience. While it's important to have clear goals and habits, being too rigid can set you up for frustration and disappointment. Allow yourself room for occasional indulgences and be prepared to adjust your strategies as needed based on changing life circumstances.

One powerful tool for building resilience is to cultivate a support network. This might include friends or family members who share your health goals, a registered dietitian who can provide professional guidance, or an online community of individuals on similar journeys. Having people to turn to for encouragement, advice, and accountability can make a significant difference in your ability to overcome obstacles and stay committed to your healthy eating goals.

It's also important to celebrate your successes, no matter how small they may seem. Each time you successfully navigate a challenging situation or resist a craving, you're building confidence and reinforcing your new habits. Take time to acknowledge these victories and use them as motivation to continue your journey.

As we conclude this chapter on overcoming obstacles and setbacks, remember that the path to healthier eating is not about perfection, but about progress. Every challenge you face and overcome makes you stronger and more capable of maintaining your healthy habits in the long run. By developing strategies to deal with cravings and emotional eating, learning to bounce back from slip-ups, and building your resilience, you're equipping yourself with the tools needed for lasting success in your nutrition journey.

As we move forward, we'll explore the important relationship between nutrition and physical activity. Understanding how these two aspects of health work together can provide additional motivation and support for your healthy eating habits. The next chapter will delve into the synergy between nutrition and exercise, offering insights on how to fuel your body effectively for different types of physical activity and how movement can enhance your overall health and wellbeing.

Chapter 16: The Role of Exercise in Healthy Eating

As we transition from our discussion on overcoming obstacles and setbacks in your healthy eating journey, it's crucial to recognize that nutrition doesn't exist in a vacuum. The food we consume is intricately linked to our physical activity, and understanding this connection can significantly enhance our overall health and well-being. In this chapter, we'll explore the synergistic relationship between nutrition and exercise, discover ways to incorporate movement into our daily lives, and learn how to properly fuel our workouts for optimal performance and recovery.

The relationship between what we eat and how we move is bidirectional and complex. Our dietary choices influence our energy levels, physical performance, and recovery, while our exercise habits can shape our nutritional needs and even our food preferences. This symbiotic relationship forms the foundation of a holistic approach to health that goes beyond simply counting calories or logging miles on a treadmill.

Let's begin by examining the synergy between nutrition and physical activity. When we engage in regular exercise, our bodies undergo numerous physiological changes. These adaptations require adequate nutritional support to be effective and sustainable. For instance, resistance training stimulates muscle protein synthesis, but without sufficient protein intake, our bodies cannot fully capitalize on this stimulus to build and repair muscle tissue. Similarly, endurance activities deplete our glycogen stores, and proper carbohydrate intake is essential for replenishing these energy reserves.

Conversely, our nutritional choices can significantly impact our exercise performance and recovery. Consuming a balanced meal containing carbohydrates and protein before a workout can provide the necessary energy and amino acids to fuel our efforts and prevent excessive muscle breakdown. Post-exercise nutrition, particularly the timing and composition of meals, plays a crucial role in replenishing energy stores, repairing damaged tissues, and promoting adaptations that lead to improved fitness over time.

Understanding this interplay allows us to make more informed decisions about both our diet and exercise habits. For example, if you're embarking on a new fitness routine, you may need to adjust your caloric intake to support increased energy expenditure. Conversely, if you're looking to lose weight, combining dietary changes with increased physical activity can lead to more sustainable results than focusing on diet alone.

Incorporating movement into our daily routines is another essential aspect of this synergy. In our increasingly sedentary world, finding ways to be more active throughout the day can have profound effects on our health and metabolism. This doesn't necessarily mean spending hours at the gym; rather, it's about making conscious choices to move more in our everyday lives.

One effective strategy is to practice "exercise snacking" – short bursts of activity spread throughout the day. This could involve taking a brisk 5-minute walk every hour, doing a set of bodyweight squats during commercial breaks while watching TV, or opting for the stairs instead of the elevator. These small habits, when consistently practiced, can accumulate to significant physical activity over time and complement our structured exercise routines.

Another approach is to seek out opportunities for active transportation. If feasible, consider walking or cycling for short trips instead of driving. Not only does this increase your daily activity level, but it also contributes to reduced carbon emissions – a win for both personal and planetary health. For those with desk jobs, standing desks or treadmill desks can be valuable tools for incorporating more movement into the workday.

It's important to note that different types of physical activity have varying effects on our bodies and, consequently, our nutritional needs. Endurance activities like long-distance running or cycling primarily rely on carbohydrates for fuel, while strength training has a greater impact on protein requirements for muscle repair and growth. Understanding these distinctions can help us tailor our nutrition to support our specific exercise goals.

For endurance athletes or those engaging in prolonged aerobic activities, carbohydrate intake becomes crucial. The body's preferred fuel source during moderate to high-intensity endurance exercise is glucose, which is stored in the muscles and liver as glycogen. Depleting these glycogen stores can lead to fatigue and decreased performance, a phenomenon often referred to as "hitting the wall" in endurance events. To prevent this, endurance athletes often practice carbohydrate loading before events and may consume easily digestible carbohydrates during prolonged activities.

On the other hand, individuals focused on strength training or bodybuilding may need to pay more attention to their protein intake. Resistance exercise creates micro-tears in muscle fibers, and adequate protein is necessary to repair this damage and stimulate muscle growth. While the exact protein requirements can vary based on factors like training intensity and individual goals, most research suggests that strength athletes benefit from slightly higher protein intakes compared to sedentary individuals.

Regardless of the type of exercise, proper hydration is paramount. Water plays a crucial role in regulating body temperature, transporting nutrients, and removing waste products. Even mild dehydration can negatively impact exercise performance and recovery. The amount of fluid needed can vary based on factors like climate, exercise intensity, and individual sweat rates, but a general guideline is to drink enough so that urine remains pale yellow.

Now, let's delve into the specifics of fueling workouts with proper nutrition. The timing of meals and snacks around exercise can significantly influence performance and recovery. While individual tolerances may vary, a general guideline is to consume a balanced meal containing carbohydrates and protein about 2-3 hours before exercise. This allows time for digestion while providing readily available energy for the workout.

For those who prefer to exercise early in the morning or can't fit in a full meal before their workout, a small, easily digestible snack about 30 minutes before exercise can be beneficial. Options might include a banana with a tablespoon of peanut butter, a small handful of dried fruit and nuts, or a smoothie made with fruit and Greek yogurt.

During prolonged exercise lasting more than 60-90 minutes, consuming carbohydrates can help maintain blood glucose levels and delay fatigue. This could be in the form of sports drinks, energy gels, or easily digestible foods like bananas or energy bars. The exact amount and timing can vary based on the individual and the activity, but a general guideline is to aim for 30-60 grams of carbohydrates per hour of exercise.

Post-exercise nutrition is equally important for recovery and adaptation. The "anabolic window" – a period immediately following exercise when the body is primed to utilize nutrients for repair and growth – has been a topic of much discussion in sports nutrition. While the importance of immediate post-exercise nutrition may have been somewhat overstated in the past, consuming a meal or snack containing both carbohydrates and protein within a couple of hours after exercise can support recovery.

A balanced post-workout meal might include a lean protein source like chicken or fish, complex carbohydrates such as brown rice or sweet potato, and plenty of vegetables for micronutrients and fiber. For those who struggle with appetite immediately after intense exercise, a protein shake or smoothie can be a convenient option to kickstart the recovery process.

It's crucial to remember that nutrition and exercise habits should be sustainable and enjoyable. While elite athletes may need to adhere to strict nutrition protocols, for most individuals, the goal should be to find a balance that supports their health and fitness goals while fitting into their lifestyle. This might mean experimenting with different meal timings, snack options, and exercise schedules to find what works best for you.

As we conclude this chapter, it's clear that exercise and nutrition are not isolated factors in our health journey, but rather interconnected elements that work together to support our overall well-being. By understanding and leveraging this synergy, we can optimize our efforts to build healthier habits and achieve our fitness goals.

In the next chapter, we'll explore the importance of mindset in achieving long-term success in our health journey. We'll discuss how developing a growth mindset about nutrition, overcoming all-or-nothing thinking, and cultivating self-compassion can significantly impact our ability to maintain healthy habits over time. This shift in perspective can be the key to transforming temporary changes into lifelong habits that support our health and happiness.

Chapter 17: Mindset Shifts for Long-Term Success

As we transition from our discussion on tracking progress and celebrating wins, it's crucial to recognize that sustainable dietary changes are as much about our mental approach as they are about the physical act of eating. In this chapter, we'll explore the pivotal role that mindset plays in achieving long-term success with our bite-sized habits approach to nutrition.

Developing a growth mindset about nutrition is the cornerstone of lasting dietary change. This concept, pioneered by psychologist Carol Dweck, posits that our abilities and intelligence can be developed through dedication and hard work. When applied to nutrition, a growth mindset allows us to view our eating habits as malleable rather than fixed. Instead of believing that we're inherently "bad" at eating healthily or that we'll never be able to resist certain foods, we can cultivate the belief that our nutritional choices and habits can improve over time with effort and persistence.

Consider the case of Sarah, a 42-year-old mother of two who had struggled with yo-yo dieting for most of her adult life. She often found herself saying things like, "I've always been a stress eater" or "I just don't have the willpower to eat healthily." These statements reflect a fixed mindset about her eating habits. However, when Sarah began to shift her perspective and embrace a growth mindset, she started to see possibilities for change. She reframed her thoughts to, "I'm learning to manage stress without turning to food" and "I'm developing the skills to make healthier choices." This shift in mindset opened the door for Sarah to approach her nutrition journey with curiosity and optimism rather than defeat and resignation.

To cultivate a growth mindset about nutrition, start by paying attention to your self-talk. When you catch yourself thinking in absolutes or making sweeping generalizations about your eating habits, pause and challenge those thoughts. Ask yourself, "Is this really true? Or is it just a belief I've held onto?" Then, reframe your thoughts in a way that acknowledges the potential for growth and improvement.

Another crucial aspect of developing a growth mindset is embracing challenges as opportunities for learning rather than viewing them as threats. When faced with a difficult nutritional choice or a setback in your healthy eating journey, try to approach it with curiosity. What can you learn from this situation? How can you use this experience to inform your future choices? This perspective allows you to see obstacles as stepping stones rather than roadblocks, fostering resilience and perseverance in your nutrition journey.

Overcoming all-or-nothing thinking is another vital mindset shift for long-term success in healthy eating. This black-and-white mentality often leads to cycles of restriction followed by overindulgence, undermining our efforts to establish sustainable eating habits. All-or-nothing thinking manifests in various ways when it comes to nutrition. You might find yourself labeling foods as "good" or "bad," believing that one unhealthy meal has ruined your entire day's efforts, or feeling that you must follow a diet plan perfectly or not at all.

Dr. Judith Beck, a prominent cognitive-behavioral therapist, explains, "All-or-nothing thinking can sabotage your efforts to eat healthily. It sets unrealistic expectations and doesn't allow for the natural fluctuations and imperfections that are part of any long-term behavior change." To combat this type of thinking, we need to embrace a more nuanced, flexible approach to nutrition.

Start by recognizing the spectrum of choices available to you rather than seeing things in binary terms. Instead of categorizing a meal as either "perfect" or "a complete failure," acknowledge that there's a wide range of options between these two extremes. Perhaps you chose a salad with grilled chicken for lunch, but also had a small piece of cake at a colleague's birthday celebration. Rather than writing off the entire day as "ruined," you can appreciate the nutritious choices you made while also allowing for moments of enjoyment and social connection.

Practicing self-compassion is another powerful tool in overcoming all-or-nothing thinking. When you do make a choice that doesn't align with your nutritional goals, resist the urge to berate yourself. Instead, treat yourself with the same kindness and understanding you would offer a friend in a similar situation.

Acknowledge that setbacks are a normal part of any change process, learn from the experience, and move forward with renewed commitment to your goals.

Cultivating self-compassion in your health journey is, in fact, the third crucial mindset shift we'll explore in this chapter. Many people approach dietary changes with a harsh, critical inner voice, believing that self-criticism will motivate them to stick to their goals. However, research consistently shows that self-compassion is far more effective in promoting long-term behavior change and overall well-being.

Dr. Kristin Neff, a pioneer in the study of self-compassion, defines it as having three components: self-kindness, common humanity, and mindfulness. In the context of our nutrition journey, self-kindness involves treating ourselves with understanding and patience when we face challenges or make mistakes. Common humanity reminds us that everyone struggles with healthy eating at times, and we're not alone in our difficulties. Mindfulness allows us to observe our thoughts and feelings about food and eating without judgment or over-identification.

Practicing self-compassion doesn't mean making excuses for unhealthy behaviors or giving up on our goals. Rather, it provides a supportive foundation from which we can make lasting changes. When we approach our nutrition journey with self-compassion, we're more likely to bounce back from setbacks, learn from our experiences, and maintain motivation over the long term.

To incorporate self-compassion into your healthy eating journey, start by becoming aware of your inner dialogue around food and eating. When you notice self-critical thoughts arising, pause and ask yourself, "Would I speak to a friend this way?" If not, try to reframe your thoughts in a more compassionate manner. For example, instead of berating yourself for overeating at dinner, you might say, "It's understandable that I ate more than I planned. I was feeling stressed and tired. What can I learn from this experience to support my health goals in the future?"

Remember, cultivating self-compassion is a skill that takes practice. Be patient with yourself as you work on developing this new mindset. Over time, you'll likely find that treating yourself with kindness and understanding not only feels better but also supports your long-term success in adopting healthier eating habits.

As we conclude our exploration of mindset shifts for long-term success, it's important to recognize that these changes don't happen overnight. Developing a growth mindset, overcoming all-or-nothing thinking, and cultivating self-compassion are ongoing practices that require patience and persistence. However, the impact of these mindset shifts on your nutrition journey can be profound, setting the stage for sustainable, positive changes in your eating habits.

In the next chapter, we'll delve into practical strategies for tracking your progress and celebrating your wins along the way. These tools will complement the mindset shifts we've discussed, providing tangible ways to reinforce your new, healthier approach to eating. By combining a supportive mindset with effective tracking methods, you'll be well-equipped to continue your journey towards lasting, positive changes in your nutrition habits.

Chapter 18: Tracking Progress and Celebrating Wins

As we near the end of our journey through bite-sized habits for transforming our diet, it's crucial to address the often-overlooked aspect of tracking progress and celebrating wins. This chapter builds upon the mindset shifts we discussed earlier, reinforcing the importance of acknowledging our achievements, no matter how small they may seem. By developing effective methods for monitoring habit changes, recognizing non-scale victories, and creating a reward system, we can sustain our motivation and continue making positive strides in our nutritional journey.

Effective methods for monitoring habit changes

Tracking our progress is essential for maintaining momentum and staying motivated on our path to better nutrition. However, it's important to approach this task with mindfulness and intention, ensuring that our tracking methods support rather than hinder our overall goals. One effective approach is to keep a detailed food journal. This doesn't mean obsessively counting calories or restricting intake, but rather noting what we eat, when we eat, and how we feel before and after meals. This practice can help us identify patterns, recognize triggers for unhealthy eating, and celebrate the positive changes we're making.

Digital apps can be valuable tools for tracking our nutritional habits. Many of these apps allow us to log meals, set reminders for healthy behaviors, and visualize our progress over time. However, it's crucial to choose an app that aligns with our personal goals and doesn't promote an unhealthy fixation on numbers. Remember, the goal is to cultivate awareness and support positive changes, not to create additional stress or anxiety around food.

Another effective method for monitoring habit changes is to use a simple habit tracker. This can be as straightforward as a calendar where we mark off each day we successfully implement a new habit, such as drinking eight glasses of water or including a serving of vegetables with each meal. The visual representation of our progress can be incredibly motivating, showing us at a glance how far we've come and encouraging us to maintain our streak.

For those who prefer a more qualitative approach, journaling can be an excellent way to track progress. By regularly reflecting on our eating habits, challenges we've faced, and successes we've experienced, we can gain valuable insights into our relationship with food and our overall well-being. This method allows us to capture nuances that might be missed by more quantitative tracking methods, such as improvements in energy levels, mood, or sleep quality that often accompany positive dietary changes.

It's worth noting that tracking methods may need to evolve as we progress on our journey. What works well in the beginning stages of habit formation may become less relevant or helpful as those habits become more ingrained. Be open to adjusting your tracking methods as needed, always keeping in mind that the ultimate goal is to support your long-term health and well-being.

Non-scale victories in nutrition

Too often, people equate success in their nutritional journey solely with the number on the scale. While weight can be one indicator of health for some individuals, it's far from the only measure of progress. In fact, focusing exclusively on weight can be counterproductive, leading to frustration, discouragement, and even unhealthy behaviors. Instead, it's essential to recognize and celebrate the many non-scale victories that come with improving our eating habits.

One significant non-scale victory is improved energy levels. As we nourish our bodies with balanced, nutrient-dense meals, many people find that they have more consistent energy throughout the day. They may notice less reliance on caffeine or sugar for quick energy boosts, and experience fewer energy crashes in the afternoon. This increased vitality can have a profound impact on overall quality of life, enabling us to engage more fully in work, hobbies, and relationships.

Another important non-scale victory is enhanced mood and mental clarity. The gut-brain connection is a growing area of research, with mounting evidence suggesting that what we eat can significantly impact our mental health and cognitive function. Many people report feeling more emotionally stable, less anxious, and better able to concentrate after improving their diet. These changes, while not visible on the scale, can dramatically improve our daily lives and overall well-being.

Improved sleep quality is another non-scale victory worth celebrating. As we adopt healthier eating habits, such as reducing late-night snacking or cutting back on caffeine, many people find that they fall asleep more easily and enjoy more restful sleep throughout the night. Given the crucial role that sleep plays in overall health, including weight management, this improvement can have far-reaching benefits.

Physical changes beyond weight loss are also important to acknowledge. Many people notice improvements in their skin's appearance, stronger nails, and healthier hair as they improve their nutrition. These changes are often reflective of improved overall health and can be a source of confidence and motivation.

Digestive improvements are another common non-scale victory. As we incorporate more fiber-rich foods and stay properly hydrated, many people experience less bloating, more regular bowel movements, and fewer digestive discomforts. These changes can significantly enhance our daily comfort and well-being.

Enhanced athletic performance is a non-scale victory that many people experience as they improve their nutrition. Whether it's being able to run a little further, lift a little heavier, or simply feeling more energetic during workouts, these improvements are tangible evidence of the positive impact of our dietary changes.

Perhaps one of the most significant non-scale victories is a healthier relationship with food. As we adopt a more balanced approach to eating, many people find that they experience less guilt around food, enjoy their meals more fully, and feel more in control of their eating habits. This shift can have profound implications for our mental health and overall quality of life.

It's crucial to regularly remind ourselves of these non-scale victories. One effective strategy is to keep a "victory journal" where we record these positive changes as we notice them. This practice not only helps us recognize our progress but also serves as a source of motivation during challenging times.

Creating a reward system for sustained motivation

While the intrinsic rewards of improved health and well-being are significant, creating an external reward system can provide additional motivation, especially in the early stages of habit formation. However, it's essential to design this system thoughtfully, ensuring that our rewards align with and support our overall health goals.

One effective approach is to create a tiered reward system, with small rewards for daily or weekly achievements and larger rewards for reaching major milestones. For example, successfully implementing a new healthy habit for a week might earn a relaxing bubble bath or an hour of guilt-free time for a favorite hobby. Maintaining that habit for a month could warrant a larger reward, such as a new cookbook or a massage.

It's crucial to choose rewards that don't undermine our nutritional goals. Food rewards, especially those that we've been trying to limit, can reinforce an unhealthy relationship with food and hinder our progress. Instead, focus on rewards that enhance our overall well-being or support our continued growth. This might include purchasing new kitchen equipment to make healthy cooking easier, signing up for a cooking class to expand our culinary skills, or investing in high-quality ingredients we might not normally splurge on.

Some people find it motivating to create a visual representation of their reward system. This could be a chart where stickers are added for each day a goal is met, with a larger reward earned after accumulating a certain number of stickers. Others might prefer a digital system, using a goal-tracking app that allows them to set and track progress towards rewards.

It's important to remember that the most sustainable motivation comes from intrinsic rewards - the genuine satisfaction and pride we feel in taking care of our health. As such, our external reward system should be designed to reinforce these intrinsic motivations rather than replace them. One way to do this is to include rewards that involve sharing our progress with others or giving back to our community. For example, reaching a major milestone might be celebrated by hosting a healthy dinner party for friends or volunteering at a local community garden.

As we progress on our journey, our reward system may need to evolve. What feels motivating in the early stages may become less exciting as our new habits become more ingrained. Be open to adjusting your rewards, always ensuring they align with your values and support your long-term health goals.

Remember, the ultimate goal of tracking progress and celebrating wins is to reinforce our commitment to health and well-being. By acknowledging our achievements, both big and small, we cultivate a positive mindset that supports long-term success. As we move forward, we'll explore how to adapt our habits as life circumstances change and continue our nutritional education, ensuring that our journey towards better health is truly lifelong.

Chapter 19: Advanced Bite-Sized Habits

As we near the end of our journey through bite-sized habits for transforming your diet, it's time to explore some more advanced concepts that can further enhance your nutritional lifestyle. These advanced habits build upon the foundation we've established throughout this book, offering new avenues for those ready to take their healthy eating practices to the next level. In this chapter, we'll delve into three powerful approaches: exploring plant-based eating, understanding the basics of intermittent fasting, and embracing the principles of intuitive eating.

Plant-based eating has gained significant popularity in recent years, and for good reason. This approach to nutrition focuses on consuming primarily or exclusively foods derived from plants, including fruits, vegetables, nuts, seeds, legumes, and whole grains. The benefits of a plant-based diet are numerous and well-documented. Research has shown that plant-based diets can lead to lower rates of heart disease, certain types of cancer, and type 2 diabetes. They are also associated with lower body weight and reduced inflammation in the body.

One of the key advantages of plant-based eating is its positive impact on the environment. Plant-based diets generally have a lower carbon footprint compared to diets heavy in animal products. By reducing our consumption of meat and dairy, we can significantly decrease our individual environmental impact. As climate change becomes an increasingly pressing issue, many people are turning to plant-based diets as a way to contribute to a more sustainable future.

Transitioning to a plant-based diet doesn't have to be an all-or-nothing proposition. In fact, adopting a flexitarian approach, where you primarily eat plant-based foods but occasionally include animal products, can be a more sustainable and realistic option for many people. This flexibility allows for easier social dining and can help prevent feelings of deprivation that might lead to abandoning the diet altogether.

When exploring plant-based eating, it's crucial to ensure you're getting all the necessary nutrients. Protein, often a concern for those new to plant-based diets, can be readily obtained from sources such as legumes, nuts, seeds, and whole grains. Foods like quinoa and soy products are complete proteins, containing all nine essential amino acids. Iron, another nutrient of concern, can be found in leafy greens, legumes, and fortified foods. Pairing iron-rich foods with vitamin C sources can enhance absorption.

Vitamin B12, primarily found in animal products, is one nutrient that requires special attention in a plant-based diet.

Supplementation or consumption of fortified foods is often necessary to meet B12 requirements. Omega-3 fatty acids, typically associated with fish, can be obtained from plant sources like flaxseeds, chia seeds, and walnuts, though some people may choose to supplement with algae-based omega-3s.

As you explore plant-based eating, remember to focus on whole, minimally processed foods. A plant-based diet centered around fruits, vegetables, whole grains, and legumes is vastly different from one reliant on processed vegan junk food. The key is to embrace the variety and richness of plant-based whole foods, experimenting with new ingredients and recipes to keep your meals exciting and satisfying.

Moving on to our second advanced habit, let's explore the basics of intermittent fasting. This eating pattern has gained considerable attention in recent years for its potential health benefits and its ability to simplify eating decisions for some individuals. Intermittent fasting is not a diet in the traditional sense, but rather an eating schedule that alternates between periods of eating and fasting.

There are several popular methods of intermittent fasting. The 16/8 method involves fasting for 16 hours and eating within an 8-hour window each day. For example, you might eat between 12 pm and 8 pm and fast from 8 pm to 12 pm the next day. Another approach is the 5:2 diet, where you eat normally for five days of the week and significantly reduce calorie intake (typically to 500-600 calories) on the other two non-consecutive days.

The potential benefits of intermittent fasting are wide-ranging. Some studies suggest it can lead to weight loss, improved insulin sensitivity, reduced inflammation, and even enhanced longevity. The mechanisms behind these benefits are still being researched, but they may be related to the metabolic switch that occurs during fasting, where the body shifts from using glucose as its primary fuel source to using fatty acids and ketone bodies.

One of the appealing aspects of intermittent fasting for many people is its simplicity. Instead of constantly thinking about what to eat, you only need to focus on when to eat. This can reduce decision fatigue and simplify meal planning. However, it's crucial to note that intermittent fasting is not suitable for everyone. Pregnant women, individuals with a history of eating disorders, and those with certain medical conditions should avoid intermittent fasting or consult with a healthcare professional before trying it.

When practicing intermittent fasting, it's essential to maintain a focus on nutrition during eating periods. The quality of your diet still matters greatly. Use your eating windows to consume nutrient-dense, whole foods that will nourish your body and keep you satisfied during fasting periods. Staying well-hydrated is also crucial, especially during fasting periods.

It's worth noting that intermittent fasting can be combined with other dietary approaches, including plant-based eating. Some individuals find that a plant-based diet complements their intermittent fasting routine well, as plant-based meals can be nutrient-dense and satisfying, helping to stave off hunger during fasting periods.

The third advanced habit we'll explore is intuitive eating. This approach represents a significant shift from traditional dieting mentalities, focusing instead on developing a healthy relationship with food and your body. Intuitive eating is based on the premise that your body knows best what it needs, and by learning to listen to and trust your body's signals, you can achieve a balanced and satisfying approach to eating.

Intuitive eating is guided by ten core principles, as outlined by dietitians Evelyn Tribole and Elyse Resch. These principles include rejecting the diet mentality, honoring your hunger, making peace with food, challenging the food police, respecting your fullness, discovering the satisfaction factor, honoring your health with gentle nutrition, coping with emotions without using food, respecting your body, and exercising for the joy of movement rather than calorie burning.

At its core, intuitive eating is about breaking free from the cycle of restrictive dieting and learning to trust your body's innate wisdom about food. This approach encourages you to eat when you're hungry and stop when you're full, to enjoy your food without guilt, and to make food choices that honor both your health and your taste preferences.

One of the key aspects of intuitive eating is learning to distinguish between physical and emotional hunger. Physical hunger is a biological signal that your body needs fuel, while emotional hunger is driven by feelings such as stress, boredom, or sadness. By becoming more attuned to these different types of hunger, you can respond more appropriately, addressing emotional needs without using food as a coping mechanism.

Intuitive eating also involves challenging ingrained beliefs about "good" and "bad" foods. Instead of labeling foods as off-limits or seeing them as rewards, intuitive eaters aim to neutralize their relationship with all foods. This doesn't mean eating junk food all the time, but rather removing the moral value from food choices and allowing yourself to enjoy all foods in moderation.

A crucial component of intuitive eating is the concept of gentle nutrition. This involves making food choices that honor your health and taste buds while making you feel good. It's about nourishing your body with nutritious foods most of the time, but also allowing for flexibility and enjoyment. Gentle nutrition recognizes that health is not just about the nutrients you consume, but also about your overall relationship with food and eating.

Adopting an intuitive eating approach can be challenging, especially for those who have a long history with dieting. It requires patience, self-compassion, and a willingness to unlearn deeply ingrained habits and beliefs about food and body image. However, many people find that intuitive eating leads to a more peaceful and satisfying relationship with food in the long run.

It's important to note that while intuitive eating can be a powerful tool for developing a healthy relationship with food, it may not be appropriate for everyone, particularly those with certain medical conditions that require specific dietary restrictions. As with any significant change to your eating habits, it's wise to consult with a healthcare professional or registered dietitian before fully embracing intuitive eating.

As we conclude our exploration of these advanced bite-sized habits, it's worth reflecting on how they might fit into your personal nutrition journey. Plant-based eating, intermittent fasting, and intuitive eating are all powerful approaches that can enhance your relationship with food and potentially improve your overall health. However, they are not one-size-fits-all solutions.

The key is to approach these advanced habits with curiosity and flexibility. Experiment with incorporating elements that resonate with you, always listening to your body and adjusting as needed. Remember, the goal is to find an approach to eating that is sustainable, enjoyable, and supports your overall health and well-being.

As we move into our final chapter, we'll discuss how to adapt your habits as life circumstances change and the importance of continuing education in nutrition. We'll also explore how you can become a role model for healthy eating, inspiring others on their own nutrition journeys. The path to lifelong healthy eating is a continuous journey of learning, adapting, and growing, and these advanced habits are just a few of the many tools available to support you along the way.

Chapter 20: Your Lifelong Nutrition Journey

As we reach the culmination of our exploration into bite-sized habits for transforming your diet, it's essential to recognize that the journey doesn't end here. In fact, this chapter marks the beginning of a lifelong commitment to nourishing your body and mind through mindful eating practices. The habits you've cultivated throughout this book are not meant to be temporary fixes, but rather the foundation for a sustainable and adaptable approach to nutrition that will serve you well into the future.

Adapting habits as life circumstances change is a crucial skill in maintaining a healthy relationship with food. Life is dynamic, and your nutritional needs and challenges will inevitably shift over time. Perhaps you're entering a new phase of life, such as starting a family or transitioning into retirement. Maybe you're facing health challenges that require dietary modifications, or you're moving to a new country with different food customs. Whatever changes come your way, the principles of bite-sized habits can be applied to navigate these transitions smoothly.

Consider the example of starting a family. The demands of pregnancy and early parenthood can significantly impact eating routines. During pregnancy, nutritional needs increase, and after the birth of a child, time for meal preparation may become scarce. In such situations, the habit of meal planning becomes even more critical. You might adapt this habit by focusing on nutrient-dense, easy-to-prepare meals that can be made in larger batches. The mindful eating practices you've developed can help you tune into your body's changing needs and ensure you're nourishing yourself adequately, even when time is limited.

Similarly, as you age, your metabolism and nutritional requirements may change. The portion control habits you've established can be adjusted to account for these shifts. You might find that you need smaller portions to maintain a healthy weight, or that you need to increase your intake of certain nutrients like calcium and vitamin D for bone health. The key is to approach these changes with the same mindful awareness and flexibility that you've cultivated throughout your journey.

Continuing education in nutrition is another vital aspect of your lifelong journey. The field of nutrition science is constantly evolving, with new research emerging regularly. Staying informed about the latest findings can help you refine your eating habits and make more informed choices. However, it's important to approach new information with a critical eye and not be swayed by every passing food trend or fad diet.

One effective way to continue your nutrition education is to follow reputable sources of information. This might include subscribing to nutrition journals, attending workshops or webinars led by registered dietitians, or following evidence-based nutrition blogs. Remember the lesson from earlier chapters about developing a growth mindset – approach new information with curiosity and openness, but also with healthy skepticism.

As you encounter new nutritional concepts, consider how they align with the principles of bite-sized habits. For instance, if you come across research suggesting benefits of a particular eating pattern, think about how you could incorporate elements of it gradually into your routine, rather than making drastic changes overnight. This approach allows you to experiment and find what works best for you without disrupting the healthy habits you've already established.

Moreover, your nutrition journey isn't just about personal growth – it's also an opportunity to positively influence those around you. As you progress in your journey, you may find yourself becoming a role model for healthy eating, whether intentionally or not. Friends, family members, or colleagues might notice the positive changes in your eating habits and approach to food, and seek your advice or inspiration.

Becoming a role model for healthy eating doesn't mean you need to be perfect or preach to others about their food choices. Instead, it's about leading by example and sharing your experiences when appropriate. You might find yourself naturally incorporating your healthy habits into social situations, such as suggesting a nutritious option when planning a group meal or demonstrating mindful eating practices at the dinner table.

If you have children, your role in shaping their relationship with food is particularly significant. By modeling balanced, mindful eating habits, you're setting a powerful example that can influence their lifelong approach to nutrition. This might involve involving them in meal planning and preparation, discussing the importance of various nutrients, or simply demonstrating a positive and relaxed attitude towards food.

Remember, being a role model also means being honest about the challenges and setbacks you face. Share not just your successes, but also how you navigate difficulties and bounce back from slip-ups. This honesty can be incredibly empowering for others who may be struggling with their own nutrition journey.

As you continue on your path, it's important to regularly reflect on your progress and reassess your goals. The SMART goal-setting techniques you learned earlier in the book can be applied periodically to ensure your nutrition goals remain aligned with your current life circumstances and values. Perhaps your initial goal was to increase your vegetable intake, and now that this has become a habit, you're ready to explore more advanced nutrition concepts like balancing macronutrients or experimenting with different eating patterns.

Reflection also involves celebrating your achievements, no matter how small they may seem. Take time to acknowledge how far you've come since you first began implementing bite-sized habits. Maybe you've completely transformed your relationship with food, or perhaps you've made small but significant improvements in specific areas of your diet. Each step forward is worthy of recognition and can serve as motivation to continue your journey.

As we conclude this chapter and the book, it's worth emphasizing that your nutrition journey is uniquely yours. While the principles and habits discussed throughout this book provide a solid foundation, the specifics of how you apply them will be shaped by your individual needs, preferences, and circumstances. Embrace this personalization and continue to experiment, learn, and grow.

Your lifelong nutrition journey is not about achieving a perfect diet or adhering to rigid rules. It's about cultivating a sustainable, flexible approach to eating that nourishes your body, supports your overall well-being, and allows you to fully enjoy the pleasures of food. By continuing to apply the concept of bite-sized habits, staying informed about nutrition, adapting to life's changes, and sharing your experiences with others, you're well-equipped to navigate the path ahead.

As you move forward from this book, carry with you the knowledge that each meal, each bite, is an opportunity to make a positive choice for your health. Your journey doesn't end here – in many ways, it's just beginning. Embrace the adventure that lies ahead, knowing that you have the tools and mindset to continue transforming your diet, one bite-sized habit at a time.

Conclusion:

As we reach the end of our journey through "Bite-Sized Habits," it's clear that transforming your diet is not about drastic changes or quick fixes. Instead, it's about embracing the power of small, consistent actions that compound over time. We've explored how tiny changes in our eating habits can lead to significant improvements in our overall health and well-being. By understanding the science of habit formation and applying it to our nutritional choices, we can create lasting change without the burnout often associated with traditional diets.

Throughout this book, we've delved into practical strategies for every aspect of healthy eating. From mindful eating and portion control to smart snacking and meal planning, each chapter has provided actionable steps to improve your relationship with food. We've learned how to navigate social situations, overcome obstacles, and celebrate our progress along the way. The importance of aligning our nutrition goals with our personal values and lifestyle has been a recurring theme, emphasizing that there's no one-size-fits-all approach to healthy eating.

One of the most crucial takeaways is the interconnectedness of our habits. We've seen how proper hydration, regular exercise, and a positive mindset all play vital roles in supporting our nutritional goals. By adopting a holistic approach to health, we set ourselves up for long-term success. The bite-sized habits approach allows us to make sustainable changes without feeling overwhelmed, gradually building a foundation for lifelong healthy eating.

As you move forward on your nutrition journey, remember that progress is not linear. There will be challenges and setbacks, but with the tools and knowledge gained from this book, you're well-equipped to overcome them. Cultivate self-compassion, embrace a growth mindset, and continue to educate yourself about nutrition. Your journey doesn't end here; it's an ongoing process of learning, adapting, and growing.

By focusing on bite-sized habits, you've taken the first steps towards a healthier, more balanced relationship with food. These small changes will ripple out into other areas of your life, influencing not just your own health but potentially inspiring those around you. As you continue to implement these habits, you'll find that healthy eating becomes less of a chore and more of a natural, enjoyable part of your daily life.

Remember, transforming your diet one meal at a time is not just about the food on your plate. It's about nourishing your body, mind, and spirit. It's about creating a lifestyle that supports your well-being and allows you to thrive. As you continue on this path, trust in the process, celebrate your victories – big and small – and embrace the journey of becoming the healthiest version of yourself.

www.ingramcontent.com/pod-product-compliance
Lightning Source LLC
Chambersburg PA
CBHW051827250726
48659CB00005B/1707